ESTABLISHING A GERIATRIC SERVICE

Establishing a Geriatric Service

Edited by Davis Coakley

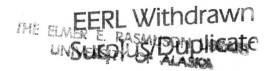

CROOM HELM
London & Canberra

© 1982 Davis Coakley
Croom Helm Ltd, 2-10 St John's Road, London SW11

British Library Cataloguing in Publication Data

Establishing a geriatric service.
   1. Aged—Medical care—Great Britain
   I. Coakley, Davis
   362.6'1'0941   HV1481.G52

   ISBN 0-7099-0700-1

Printed and bound in Great Britain
by Billing and Sons Limited
Guildford, London, Oxford, Worcester

CONTENTS

Acknowledgements

ACKNOWLEDGEMENTS

I wish to thank the authors whose experience and expertise have made this book possible. I would also like to thank my wife, Mary, who gave me invaluable help and encouragement whilst preparing the book for publication. Finally I would like to thank Michele Kilkenny for her secretarial assistance.

Davis Coakley
Dublin

1 INTRODUCTION: THE ELEMENTS OF A GERIATRIC SERVICE

D. Coakley

Industrialised countries have experienced a dramatic increase in the relative as well as the absolute number of people aged 65 or over in their populations. In most of these countries the proportion of the population over the age of 65 is greater than 10 per cent. Butler (1979) has aptly described this phenomenon as 'The Graying of Nations'. These demographic changes have placed considerable strain on health services, as the elderly are major users of a nation's health resources.

A Legacy of Deprivation

It would be wrong to believe that care of the elderly patient was adequate before these demographic changes occurred. In Britain their needs were often 'met' by the waiting list for the workhouse infirmary. These institutions had such a bad reputation that only those in really dire straits would contemplate seeking admission. Institutions such as these were unable to cope with the needs of the rapidly expanding elderly population. Many of the patients were not properly assessed on or before admission, treatable illness was not diagnosed and, as a result, a considerable number of the patients who lived permanently in these institutions were inappropriately placed.

Calls for Reform

The inadequacies of this custodial approach to the problems of the elderly were becoming more and more apparent. Numerous individuals and investigating commissions called for reform. In a report on the facilities for the elderly in the Birmingham region in 1947, Sir Arthur Thompson stated that the first step must be the establishment of wards in general hospitals and particularly in teaching hospitals in order to restore the study of the aged and the chronic sick to the common stream of medical activity (Nagley, 1972). However, the radical reforms which were to change the nature of the care of the elderly were already underway when Thompson completed his report.

A Geriatric Service

In 1935 Dr Marjorie Warren took over 874 beds in a workhouse infirmary associated with the West Middlesex Hospital, London, and by 1948 she had developed a compact efficient service with 200 beds. Dr Warren accomplished this by assessing the needs of each patient and then instigating appropriate forms of treatment and rehabilitation. With this approach many patients previously thought to be beyond remedy subsequently left hospital. On the basis of her experience Dr Warren suggested that a geriatric service should be established which would be responsible for the acute or short-term elderly sick as well as the long-term elderly sick. The proposed service should be based in a general hospital ward unit reserved exclusively for elderly patients. In these wards patients would have appropriate investigations, treatment and rehabilitation to enable them to be discharged eventually to their own homes or to other appropriate accommodation (Warren, 1943).

Domiciliary Assessment

At about the same time as Warren was formulating the above concepts, Bluestone was pioneering a home care programme at the Montefiore Hospital in New York. This programme demonstrated that many patients who would otherwise have been admitted to an institution could receive excellent care at home. The initial team consisted of a doctor, nurse and social worker. Later, physiotherapists, speech therapists and occupational therapists joined the programme. Although the scheme generated considerable interest in the United States, the growth of similar units there has been slow for a number of reasons (Rossman and Burnside, 1975). Bluestone's system was modified and adapted to the English scene by Brooke at Carshalton in Surrey. Brooke began to carry out home assessments on all the patients referred to his unit. He identified their needs, both medical and social, and he then planned appropriately (Nagley, 1972). Domiciliary assessment was subsequently adopted by others throughout the country and it is still an important aspect of the work of many geriatric units today (Chapter 3).

The Day Hospital

The day hospital is essentially a hospital without beds and this concept was first developed within the psychiatric services of the USSR. It was introduced as part of the geriatric service in the United Kingdom at Oxford in 1958, and like domiciliary visiting its success ensured that it quickly became a standard feature of most services throughout the country (Chapter 4). Day hospitals have been slow to develop in the United States, partly because of unsustained financial support. However, there has been increased interest in them in recent years as health planners look for alternatives to institutionalisation.

Teamwork

With the inception of the National Health Service geriatric medicine was recognised as a specialty in Britain. Departments were developed throughout the country around the consultant and his staff. The emphasis on rehabilitation and discharge to the community meant that these consultants had to build up close relationships with caring agencies in the community. In fact it almost invariably meant that the consultants had to play an active part in the planning and development of these agencies.

The consultants also had to encourage a multidisciplinary approach to the problems of patients admitted to their unit. The frail elderly usually have multiple problems and they need the services of different professional groups such as occupational therapists, physiotherapists and social workers. Ensuring that the team works efficiently, so that patients derive most benefit, is a skilful task demanding many attributes from the team leader (Chapter 8). Multidisciplinary ward rounds or case conferences with representatives from the community attending are regular features of most modern geriatric units.

Community Care

Parallel with the developments in hospital care there have been significant improvements in the community care of the elderly sick during the past 30 years. The family doctor is central to most of these improvements as he deals with most of the health problems of the elderly in the community. Many areas now have centres with primary health care teams (Chapter 2). When a patient needs the special skills of a physician in geriatric medicine the family doctor can call on the services of his local consultant. Close co-operation between the hospital-based consultant and the family doctor ensures optimum care for the patient as well as optimum use of resources.

In Britain social services and amenities for the elderly have also improved considerably and both hospital and family doctors can now rely on a range of services for dependent patients living at home (Chapter 9). In the United States, however, except for home health services under Medicare, it has not been government policy to make generally available the social and health services that are intended to make it possible for the frail elderly to remain at home if they so desire. The availability of services such as meals-on-wheels, home help, day care centres and similar supportive services depends very much on where the old person lives (Ball, 1977).

Interdisciplinary Co-operation

Dementia is one of the major determinants of breakdown leading to institutional care (Arie, 1977). In recent years more positive and constructive approaches to the problems of demented patients and their relatives have emerged in the United Kingdom. There has been closer co-operation between psychiatrists and physicians involved in the care of the elderly and the result has been a much more efficient service (Chapter 10).

Another example of the value of good interdisciplinary co-operation is the excellent orthopaedic services which have developed in areas where the surgical and geriatric teams work closely together (Chapter 11). There is scope for this type of co-operation in other areas, for example the treatment of elderly patients with conditions such as stroke, vascular disease or urological problems.

Research and Teaching

In geriatric medicine students are exposed in a practical way to the ideal of modern medical education, whole-person-medicine, where the physical, social and psychological needs of patients are considered of equal importance. Fostering positive attitudes towards elderly patients involves teaching modern concepts to a wide range of different professional groups including nurses, doctors, social workers, ambulance personnel, physiotherapists, occupational and diversional therapists, etc. Studies in the United States have shown that medical student interest in geriatric medicine diminishes as students progress through the under-graduate years (Institute of Medicine, 1978). However, the development of negative attitudes was not inevitable and the presence of respected faculty role models fostered positive attitudes. In the United Kingdom over 50 per cent of the medical schools now have academic units of geriatric medicine (Chapter 14). Already research groups within geriatric medicine have been active in further studies of subjects such as stroke, falls, incontinence, bone disease and nutrition (Isaacs, 1978). There is particular scope for interdisciplinary and interdepartmental co-operation in developing research in geriatric medicine.

Planning and Monitoring Progress

Those who have developed a good service or those who are striving to build one cannot afford to be complacent about their achievements. The service should be assessed regularly both in terms of efficiency and in terms of the quality of life of the patients within the service (Chapter 7). The computer can be used to advantage both to monitor and plan for the elderly (Chapter 12). Opportunities to improve the design of wards so that the environment is as pleasant as possible for both staff and patients should be taken whenever possible (Chapter 5). Equipment should be reviewed regularly and the staff should be familiar with the wide range of aids which is available for the disabled (Chapter 6).

The Elderly and Modern Technology

Elderly patients can benefit greatly from the advance in medical technology. The new non-invasive methods of investigation are a considerable advantage to doctors when confronted with the multiple pathology of the older patient. Advances in surgery and anaesthesia have made procedures much safer. There have been considerable advances also in the treatment of acute illness in old age (Coakley, 1981) and physicians caring for elderly patients should be in a position to avail themselves of these advances for the benefit of their patients. It is for these reasons that the British Geriatrics Society has insisted that at least one-third and preferably one-half of all geriatric beds in an area should be in a general hospital.

In a number of chapters in this book the point is made that the nature of the service in any particular area is closely related to the quality and enthusiasm of the physician who has established the service. Few could argue with the fact that much has been achieved over the past 30 years. However, there is still much to be accomplished today and many physicians face daunting problems, both in Britain and in other countries, with the same zeal as the early pioneers in the field. This book has been written in the hope of helping these physicians and their colleagues in administration, nursing and paramedical disciplines in their determination to develop an excellent service for elderly patients. Some of the chapters have been written by doctors who have established units of international renown. Other chapters describe the practical difficulties encountered by younger doctors and their colleagues when establishing or developing different aspects of a geriatric service today. While in the main the book draws on British experience (except specifically in Chapter 13), it is hoped that readers in other countries will be able to learn from both our successes and mistakes. A glossary of terms relating to the UK health service is given towards the end of the book for readers unfamiliar with such terms.

References

Arie, T. (1977). 'Issues in the Psychiatric Care of the Elderly', in *Care of the Elderly*. A.N. Exton-Smith and J.G. Evans (eds.), Academic Press, London and Grune and Stratton, New York

Ball, R.M. (1977). 'United States Policy toward the Elderly', in *Care of the Elderly*. A.W. Exton-Smith and J.G. Evans (eds.). Academic Press, London, and Grune and Stratton, New York

Butler, R.N. (1979). *The Graying of Nations: Creative Responses.* Age Concern, London

Coakley, D. (ed.) (1981). *Acute Geriatric Medicine.* Croom Helm, London; PSG, Littleton, Mass.

Institute of Medicine (1978). *Ageing and Medical Education.* National Academy of Sciences, Washington

Isaacs, B. (1978). *Recent Advances in Geriatric Medicine.* Churchill Livingstone, London and New York

Nagley, L. (1972). 'In the Beginning', in *Symposia on Geriatric Medicine*, Vol. 1. R.D.T. Cape (ed.), West Midland Institute of Geriatric Medicine and Gerontology, Birmingham

Rossman, L. and Burnside, I.M. (1975). 'The United States of America', in *Geriatric Care in Advanced Societies.* J.C. Brocklehurst (ed.). M.T.P. Lancaster; University Park Press, Baltimore

Warren, M.W. (1943). 'A Case for treating chronic sick in blocks in a general hospital'. *British Medical Journal*, V, 822-3.

2 ASSESSING THE NEED OF AN AREA

M.R.P. Hall

Most geriatric services have arisen to meet a need which already existed. This need might have had a medical, social or mental bias so that no blueprint exists that can be taken and superimposed to meet the needs of the elderly population living in a specific area. This is probably just as well, since it is very unlikely that any two areas will be similar, for each will inevitably have its own particular customs and characteristics. The type of service which exists or needs to be provided will depend on many factors which may be traditional, social, religious, economic or political and may be influenced by external factors such as climate. To try and superimpose some Western systems in an Eastern community would probably lead to failure.

Many services, like 'TOPSY', have 'just growed', being influenced in their growth by various entrepreneurs who by their vision, drive and enthusiasm have developed a method of care which may or may not be applicable to another service in a different community. Examples of such schemes are 'Home for the weekend, back on Monday' (Parnell and Naylor, 1973) and 'Six weeks in, six weeks out' (DeLargy, 1957), while others are dealt with in greater detail in later chapters of this book (cf. Chapters 3 and 11). In order to establish a satisfactory geriatric service for a specific area one must look closely at the needs of that area and assess how the existing resources already meet that need. Having done this one can then decide what additional resources must be provided to meet the need or whether existing resources can be adapted.

The provision of an efficient health care service for the elderly (geriatric service) depends upon the co-operation and collaboration of many agencies and the more complex the social structure, the more agencies and disciplines, and therefore people, may become involved in the provision of health care. Consequently it becomes harder to assess the need and then to meet the need. In the simplest society based on agriculture, in which the older person continues to have a role of importance to that society, the major need is likely to be that of food and the medical service will probably have little difficulty in meeting the health need. In an advanced post-industrial society (Dumazedier,

1972), with a small nuclear family which may need to move in search of work leaving the elderly unsupported yet with high expectations of the welfare state, the solution to their problems is much more difficult.

'Needs' and 'Wants'

The demands of the elderly themselves and of their relatives can clearly be defined as 'wants'. These are not the same as 'needs' which may be defined as those 'wants' which are considered necessary by an observer. The extent or amount of 'need' will depend on the bias of the observer and may differ from the expressed 'want' of the individual. While 'needs' and 'wants' are sometimes appropriate, compromise is often necessary to decide what level of demand can reasonably be met or what alternatives may be acceptable.

Obviously the level of demand that can be met will depend on the resources available and how they are disposed. Little evidence, however, exists with regard to the best mix of resources necessary to meet the maximum demand. For example, Wager (1972) concluded that there was little difference in cost when intensive domiciliary care was compared to residential care. However Opit (1977) found that in 5 per cent of his sample, home care was proving more expensive than hospital care. The decision therefore whether to develop community services as opposed to residential services or hospital services may well depend on the attitudes of society. Some societies seem to have developed a tradition whereby people move into housing complexes which are designed to cater for the retired or nearly retired person and in which they can continue to live into true old age, cf. The Netherlands (Coleman, 1975). It is wrong, therefore, to advocate one type of care as being superior to another and it would also seem wrong in the light of our present knowledge to impose a particular mix of resources as a 'best buy' solution. What, however, is certain is that whatever the society or area in question, a mix of resources will be necessary to provide the best possible solution to meet the needs of the elderly within the defined area under consideration. As Irvine (1980) has pointed out, calculations of the cost of all the resources, including family manpower, needed to keep disabled elderly people at home are difficult and their validity doubtful: for the resources available in any society are finite and manpower is as important as money. All the advanced Western societies contain an increasing proportion of elderly and even the wealthiest are having to face the fact that even the provision of 70 residential/nursing home places/1,000 elderly is no longer an adequate solution to their problem.

How then can the needs of an area be assessed so that a comprehensive geriatric service can be established? In order to do this, we first need to define the objectives of our geriatric service, secondly to define the basic needs of the elderly, thirdly to prepare a conspectus of services currently available in the area for the care of the elderly and fourthly to determine the levels of need and define the major requirements at each level, i.e. in the community, for residential care and housing, and from the hospital service.

Objectives of a 'Geriatric' Service

In their report, a working party set up by the Wessex Regional Hospital Board in 1972 agreed that the aims of the services for the elderly could be stated in the following terms:

> Through the combined agency of all who are engaged in the delivery of care:
> (a) To provide medical and social care which will enable the elderly to participate in as many spheres of life as they are able, whether at home, in residential or in hospital care.
> (b) To encourage the active co-operation of families with elderly dependent relatives and to ensure their relief from excessive burdens of care.
> (c) To provide clinical treatment.
> (d) To care for the dying adequately and with sensitivity.

These aims imply that the service will be a health service as well as an illness service. Moreover, if it is really to relieve relatives of burdens of care and provide clinical treatment then it must be a 'crisis' orientated service capable of arranging immediate admission. To fulfil these aims the service must operate at a community level as well as have appropriate hospital resources such as beds, outpatient clinics, etc.

Attitudes Towards the Needs of the Elderly

The needs of the elderly are frequently only seen from a negative viewpoint. This has been described (Hall *et al.*, 1978) as the negative health

cycle (Figure 2.1) and it is easy to understand how this view gains
credence. Attitudes towards the elderly must also be taken into account

Figure 2.1: The Negative Health Cycle: A Vicious Circle of Ill Health in the Elderly

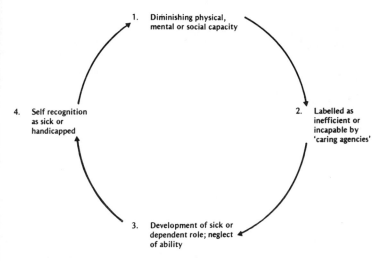

1. Diminishing physical, mental or social capacity
2. Labelled as inefficient or incapable by 'caring agencies'
3. Development of sick or dependent role; neglect of ability
4. Self recognition as sick or handicapped

when assessing the need of an area. Butler (1969) has drawn attention
to the bigotry associated with Ageism and if such attitudes exist then
the reversal of a negative health cycle (Figure 2.2) will become much
more difficult. Figure 2.2 depicts the social and health system which is
necessary for positive health in the elderly. As can be seen, the health
input is relatively small and for an old person, as for any other person,
to be able to lead a comfortable, active existence, adequately clothed,
fed, housed and supported in the community, with a continuing role
in society and the opportunity to continue to develop as an individual
should he so wish it, requires considerable resources and organisation.

Conspectus of Services

If the scheme shown in Figure 2.2 is accepted as a system within which
all the possible needs of the elderly can be met, then any inventory or
conspectus of services must go far beyond a list of what is provided by
social services and must consider housing provision, transport services
of all types, adult educational activities, employment schemes for the

Figure 2.2: The Positive Health Cycle: The Maintenance of Good Health in the Elderly

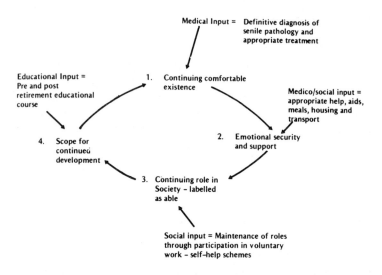

elderly, leisure activities for the elderly such as 'health and fun' clubs, the role played by voluntary organisations and privately-run organisations, some of which may be profit making, and finally the local political scene which may well change from time to time. In drawing up such an inventory it is useful to have a checklist and an example is given in Appendix A to this chapter.

Levels of Need and Requirements: In the Community

Information Services

Perhaps the most important need of all for the elderly is to know what is available so that if they then have a need they are able to state it without loss of pride to the right person. This means that the requirement is for an information service staffed by people who are sensitive to the elderly person's need and which can enable the elderly person to link with the appropriate resource. In Britain the Citizens' Advice Bureau performs this service for all age groups. Social service departments may provide an information service through their area offices and voluntary groups such as Age Concern will often run specific information centres for the elderly. Information in pamphlet or booklet form is also usually available in local public libraries and may be posted at the time of retirement with the individual's pension book. Age Concern (England) publishes a considerable amount of material containing vital information for the elderly, the chief amongst these being 'Your Rights', which is updated yearly.

General Practitioner and Community Health Services

Screening and Prevention. The elderly need to be given guidance on recognising loss of function and must be encouraged to seek advice early. The early detection and prevention of disease in the elderly has been excellently reviewed by Anderson (1978). It is well recognised that a large amount of 'unreported illness' (Williamson, 1966 and Williamson *et al.*, 1966) exists amongst old people and many surveys have confirmed this in different parts of the world (Andrews *et al.*, 1971; Ruikka, 1971; Schwenger, 1971; Akhtar *et al.*, 1973). One of the problems is how to persuade the elderly to recognise and report their disability. The GP (family doctor) and his attached health visitor (Chapter 9) are the natural focus to whom the elderly should report and the well-organised practice team will know about most of their elderly patients, particularly those at risk. General practice record systems need to be specifically organised to achieve this. Computerisation of medical records may aid this but a simple scheme using a specially designed record card has recently been tried with some success (Munday and Rowe, 1979).

Essential to any practice screening programme is first an age/sex register and secondly commitment of the team to the programme. Age/sex registers are by no means universal and family practitioner committees may be reluctant, or even refuse, to provide this. Many GPs are still unconvinced of the value of screening on the grounds that those in need are brought to their notice and those who are not known do not need any attention. There is certainly some evidence to support this but the surveys already quoted suggest that the overall standard of practice is not so high. It may be that the presence or absence of an age/sex register is the most significant pointer towards a high standard of practice.

Other schemes which will help the elderly to recognise and report their disabilities can also be devised. The Rutherglen Experiment (Anderson and Cowan, 1955) was started in a public health clinic and similar 'clinics' for the elderly have been established. These may be held by general practitioners themselves in their own premises. Health visitors and nurses can be used to visit the elderly in their homes and it has been shown that the use of structured questionnaires can be helpful in uncovering physical illness.

Family Practitioner Service. A further need of the elderly is to be able to receive medical treatment and advice when physical and mental problems appear. This forms a major part of the work of the general practitioner and the nurses attached to his team. This integration of medical and nursing disciplines has gradually developed within the National Health Service (NHS) in the United Kingdom and represents the foundation upon which a good geriatric service can be built, for without good medical and nursing care in the home no geriatric service will be able to fulfil its aim. In countries where family medical and nursing services are not as closely integrated as in the NHS, the development of a geriatric service may prove difficult.

A basic requirement, therefore, for a good geriatric service is an excellent family medical service which includes the nurse and the health visitor (or other 'preventive' agency) and their supporting services (see Chapter 9). These will include a bath attendant service, a home chiropody service, a laundry service and a nursing and home aids service which will provide 'on demand' all necessary aids (e.g. commodes, wheelchairs, etc.) including appropriate home adaptations (Hall, 1980). A night nursing or attendant service needs to be an integral part of the area's home nursing service. This family medical service will need to be supported by the hospital-based geriatric medical team. This can be done on an 'ad hoc' consultative basis, patients being seen by a member of the hospital team in their own home (domiciliary consultation) or being referred to the hospital geriatric outpatient clinic. Another way is for a senior member of the hospital team to hold a regular consultation clinic at the family doctor's premises. This may be justifiable when family doctors work in groups (group practice) or from a health centre which services a defined geographical area (MacLennan and Hall, 1980). The periodicity at which such clinics are held would depend on the size of the population served, e.g. monthly for a population of 20-25,000.

Another requirement is support from the remedial professions and both physiotherapists and occupational therapists have an important role to play in helping to restore mobility and function after a period of illness. The speech therapist too may be equally important in the case of the 'stroke' patient.

Community Medicine. The community physician and his team have a most important part to play in organising some of these supporting services as well as developing collaboration with social services and monitoring the delivery of health care to the elderly. It is also their responsibility to develop health education programmes and some of these should be directed towards the elderly. The hospital geriatric team should play a prime part in these educational activities, not only with regard to the laity. They should also organise and be involved with professional training for all involved in the health professions, whether they be students in training, qualified or unqualified. Bridging the interface between health and social services is perhaps the major task for the community physician and in many districts in the NHS one of the medical members of his team will be allocated a special role to assist with the establishment of good services for the elderly. This is in line with the recommendations of the British Medical Association's (BMA) report (1976).

Other Professional Services. Many of the disabling concomitants of old age are associated with deterioration in the special senses, sight, hearing, smell and taste. These can lead to isolation, loneliness, subnutrition and in due course physical and mental illness. About 30 per cent of the elderly have hearing difficulty and almost as many have visual problems. The presence of efficient audiological and ophthalmic services is obviously important. The attitudes of some professionals in these fields are often prejudiced so that the older person may not be considered worthy of an appropriate service. The finding of several unused and, often, useless hearing aids in an old person's house would seem to support this view. However, if hearing therapists are used then the patient may be trained to lip-read as well as use the hearing aid successfully. Unfortunately, there are only a few such therapists in the NHS, though more posts are being created. It is important to realise that the elderly can learn new things and techniques as long as their intellect is preserved intact. Consequently, age itself should never be considered a barrier to learning new skills and even braille can be learned.

Dental services for the elderly are obviously important. At present they tend to be a neglected part of the service, though the elderly are still treated by the dental practitioner services and special dental services may be provided within the hospital geriatric service.

Social Services

Departments of social services obviously play a major part in the care of the elderly. Many of the supporting services necessary to meet the needs of old people in their own homes are provided by the social service departments of the local civic authorities in the UK. Many elderly need guidance on how to cope with the problems of isolation and loneliness. Social workers assess need and then allocate the appropriate resource.

Day centres, day clubs, holiday admissions to residential homes, good neighbour schemes, street warden schemes and neighbourhood care are all schemes which can be developed by social services departments, often by encouraging their development by voluntary organisations (Chapter 9). Referral to one of these facilities will often alleviate the individual's problem. With the increasing numbers of frail elderly the need for day centres or day care centres is becoming more important.

Nutrition of the elderly is important and though surveys (DHSS, 1979) have shown that the incidence of subnutrition overall is only 7 per cent, it is twice as large in the over 80s and is particularly associated with medical and social 'risk' factors. Without the 'meals-on-wheels' service and the lunch clubs which are provided by social services there is no doubt that much more subnutrition would be seen. Some authorities have also experimented with extending neighbourhood schemes to provide food for those who need it as well as company and help in the home (Bytheway, 1980).

A good home help service is essential if the aged (over 80 years) and other elderly disabled are to maintain reasonable standards of cleanliness and tidiness in their homes. There were 6.5 home helps per 1,000 elderly in 1975 in the UK (Bytheway, 1980) but the suggested DHSS 'norm' is 12/1,000, as shown in Table 2.1.

Table 2.1: Some 'Norms' Suggested for the Elderly, Social Service Provision (HM 35/72)

Social work	50-60 per 100,000 population
Home help	12/1,000 aged 65 years or more
Mobile meals	200/1,000 aged 65 years or more
Day centres	50 places per 100,000 total population
Residential homes	25 places per 1,000 aged 65 years or more

The home help service can, however, be supplemented by good neighbour schemes and neighbourhood care schemes. The former are primarily run by voluntary agencies or individuals, albeit sponsored by local authorities, while the latter are promoted by local authorities and families or individuals are paid to 'foster' or provide some form of care for old people who might otherwise be admitted to residential care.

In addition to the provision of these supportive services the social services department also has the responsibility of providing many of the aids necessary for the elderly (e.g. commodes, etc.). There would seem to be considerable overlap with health services in this field and the development of a joint scheme is clearly indicated (Robertson and Haines, 1977).

Preparation for Retirement, Further Education and Occupation

The elderly have three main needs in this field. The first is to receive advice before retirement on how to prepare and adapt. The second is to have the opportunity to continue to work if they so desire. The third is to be able to develop activities and new interests if they so wish.

To have a successful retirement means that you need good health, money and a continuing role in society that labels you as able. In order to achieve this, retirement needs to be planned and it is almost never too early to begin to teach people about ageing and the problems that may be encountered. Consequently, a good geriatric service needs to be involved in retirement education and should encourage the local education department to run pre-retirement courses. Other bodies, such as the workers' education association, private firms and organisations, should be encouraged to do this and adult education departments in universities can also participate and stimulate this sort of education.

Attitudes of the young and the community may be altered if ageing is taught as a subject at school age. The young and the old can also become involved with one another's activities in a variety of ways, for instance through joint hobbies, clubs and voluntary activities. This type of collaboration often gives the elderly a role in life.

Similarly the elderly should be given work opportunities. Some firms, for instance, run special workplaces for their retired workers, with union backing. Some labour exchanges also keep a roster of elderly who want to do certain types of work which others may not wish to do, e.g. traffic crossing supervisors, gardening, etc. Adult educational opportunities are also important to help the elderly to learn new skills. However, it should be remembered that although the elderly can learn, as the work done at the University of Queensland has shown, teaching methods need to be different with a slower pace, more repetition, group work and self testing.

Housing and Residential Needs

As soon as disability occurs the initial need will be for home adaptations and aids. This need and the requirement to fulfil it has already been mentioned. Nevertheless, this need is often tardily met and demarcation disputes between various authorities often occur. In some services in other countries, e.g. Victoria, Australia, appropriate craftsmen can be sent from the hospital geriatric service into the patient's home so that adaptations can be tailored by the therapists to the individual patient's need.

If housing is unsuitable, and much of the housing occupied by the elderly is old and in disrepair, then good ordinary housing is the first essential. This may be publicly or privately owned housing, or run by a voluntary housing association, who can often get grants from government to develop housing for the elderly. Housing should take the form of flats, ground floor or with lifts, or bungalows, and should be sited as near to community facilities such as shops, pubs, churches, bus stops as possible. It should be integrated within ordinary housing for younger people, though some specially grouped dwellings for the elderly in quieter conclaves will also be necessary.

Sheltered Housing. If disability is great, then sheltered housing schemes with an attached warden are essential (Chapter 9). Moreover if additional warden support is provided so that 24 hour, 7 day per week cover is provided, then extremely disabled elderly may be cared for. The Kinloss Court experiment in Southampton (England) is of this nature and assessment of residents has shown that they are as disabled as the elderly in local authority residential homes (Hampshire Social Services, 1979).

There is no doubt that good housing makes home care for the elderly easier. This particularly applies to the elderly disabled and housing should be designed and built so that wheelchair use and access is easy. Adequate provision of sheltered housing schemes can go a long way towards relieving the burden on both local authority residential home places and hospital beds. The exact number of sheltered housing places appropriate for an elderly population has yet to be defined. The Scottish Development Department has suggested 25 places per 1,000 over 65 years, while Townsend (1962) has suggested 50 places. Experience would suggest that this latter figure is probably a minimum. Beverfelt (1980) reported that a survey in Norway in 1974 showed that less than 4 per cent of the elderly lived in special flats and commented that waiting lists suggested an extensive unmet need. In the same year (1974) the Netherlands had 120,000 such dwellings in which 13 per cent of the elderly lived. The goal was to increase this proportion to 25 per cent by 1985 (Van Zonneveld, 1980).

The Southampton study quoted above has underlined the need for close collaboration between statutory authorities, e.g. health, social services and housing, not only in the planning of residential accommodation but also in the placement of people within this. Individuals' needs change with time and there should be free and easy movement between different types of accommodation with trials by the client so that an appropriate choice may be made for the benefit of all concerned.

Residential Homes. When sheltered housing is inappropriate, then the client may need to be looked after in some form of residential accommodation which will provide a considerable amount of support (Chapter 9). The individual will, in this stage, be so incapacitated that he/she is unable to live even in sheltered housing, but is not so disabled as to need a permanent hospital or nursing home bed. In the UK the local authority social services departments are responsible for the provision of residential homes staffed by trained care attendants. The suggested DHSS 'norm' is 25 places per 1,000 aged 65 years or more and this includes some places for the elderly severely mentally infirm (ESMI) (Table 2.1).

In addition to this social service provision, the local authority social services departments are responsible for licensing rest homes for the elderly which are run by private individuals or by voluntary organisations like the Abbeyfield Society. Consequently, in assessing the profile of any area, it is necessary to consider the part played by these other resources in meeting needs.

Recent surveys of homes run by the local authority have revealed an increasing number of very frail and aged elderly, some of whom are unsuitable for such homes because their care places too heavy a burden on the staff. Such reviews (Dodd *et al.*, 1980) show that while misplacement is not excessive (about 6 per cent), it may be detrimental to the proper running of a home and this fact should be remembered when the staffing structure of residential homes is considered. This may be particularly important in view of the likely increase in the number of elderly aged 75 years or more.

It is clear that local authority residential homes form an essential part of the geriatric service and places must be used as effectively as possible. Most authorities now reserve a proportion of places for short-term relief, similar to the 'holiday' relief provided in the hospital service. This means that they nearly always have the ability to meet 'short-term crisis' situations and admit people who don't appear to need medical care. However, frequently the apparent 'social crisis' has an underlying physical or mental background and close collaboration between the GP responsible for such patients and the hospital geriatric and psychogeriatric service is essential in order to reduce the risk of misplacement. Moreover, selection of suitable residents poses problems and a health service representative on the selection panel is essential. Many panels agree to distribute vacancies according to a preset plan, e.g. every third vacancy goes to a patient in hospital who can only be discharged to a residential home. A recent study (Spackman, 1980) suggests that this may be an inappropriate balance and that a greater proportion of vacancies should be given to the hospital population. However, this may only indicate a difference in resources and their utilisation between areas and the warning, given at the introduction of this chapter concerning the difficulty of copying policies and methods of practice, must be repeated. Nevertheless, policy with regard to this aspect of practice should be monitored in all areas and adjusted as required.

The liaison between the statutory authorities must be good. There must also be a good relationship between the geriatric service and individuals who run private homes as well as with voluntary organisations which are involved in this field. In many parts of the world it is the voluntary organisations which provide the bulk of the residential care. They are often backed by religious organisations. The statutory geriatric service should aim at providing support to all those people who cater for this need, so that the quality of life provided for the elderly is of the highest order.

The Hospital Service. In the UK this service is provided by the NHS and although many elderly may be treated on a short-term basis by private medicine, as yet no private geriatric hospitals exist. There are, however, many nursing homes, licensed by the health authority and run either by religious nursing orders or private individuals. The contribution that these can make to the overall service must be borne in mind.

So far this chapter has concentrated on the community role that should be played by any good geriatric service. Indeed if they are to be successful in providing a comprehensive service for the health care of the elderly, the geriatric and psychogeriatric services must concentrate on supporting the community elements described and must help to organise them through the area or district health care planning team for the elderly. By doing this they can stimulate early referral of patients by general practitioners and by appropriate treatment maintain function at a high level. They can also educate all involved with the elderly concerning the efficacy of geriatric medicine and psychiatry.

Health Care Planning Team

The various elements involved in the care of the elderly can only work effectively and efficiently if they collaborate. In order to do this the individual groups need to understand each other's policies, what resources each have, what each other's difficulties and deficiencies are, and they must plan to make the best use of resources. Dialogue between groups of workers is necessary to achieve this and an effective health care planning team is essential. Each group concerned with the care of the elderly should be represented on this team so that each can put forward his view and report back to his group. The team should be kept as small as possible and dialogue should be aimed at identifying deficiencies and making short- and long-term plans to correct these. Representatives should therefore be senior members of their groups and should be able to make accurate judgements of the appropriateness of actions which their groups may need to take to improve situations.

Levels of Need and Requirements: Geriatric and Psychogeriatric Services

Geriatric Medical Services

The hospital unit and the facilities it requires together with its operational policy are discussed in detail in other chapters. Its role is to meet the need for an expert opinion at an early stage of incapacity and to give treatment for that incapacity with or without admission to hospital. If admission to hospital is indicated then the patient will need access to all diagnostic facilities and specialist services. If urgent admission is required then beds need to be available. Since recovery from illness in old age is often slow, continuing treatment will need to be in active rehabilitation wards which are geared to meet the needs of the elderly. Some patients will prove irremediable and require longer rehabilitation programmes or even permanent long-term care in accommodation which is suited to their needs. Where relatives bear a heavy nursing or caring load at home, intermittent admissions may be necessary to relieve these burdens of care. Some patients will need admission for the terminal period of their illness.

To meet these needs the geriatric medical service has the following requirements:

To run a domiciliary consultation service and support the family doctor in his home care of the patient (hospital at home service).
To hold outpatient clinics.
To have day hospital facilities.
To have acute beds in the district general hospital.
To have beds for active short-term (approx. 3 months) rehabilitation.
To have beds for intermittent admission, holiday relief, longer-term rehabilitation, long stay care and terminal care.

In the NHS it has been suggested that the resources shown in Table 2.2 should be provided to meet these requirements. These 'norms' can be queried and many surveys suggest that the bed norm in particular is deficient. This, however, is not borne out by the trends which have taken

Table 2.2: Geriatric Service Norms (DS329/71 and HM72/71)

HOSPITAL BEDS
    Medical 10 per 1,000 aged 65 years or more
    Psychiatric 2.5-3 per 1,000 aged 65 years or more
    Medical/Psychiatric Assessment 10-20 per 250,000 total population
DAY HOSPITAL PLACES
    Medical 2 per 1,000 aged 65 years or more
    Psychiatric 2-3 per 1,000 aged 65 years or more

place in geriatric medicine over the past 20 years within the UK and Slattery and Bourne (1979) have argued that a lower bed 'norm' may be appropriate if length of patient stay continues to fall and discharge rates rise. It can be argued that this is likely to happen if geriatric medical services adopt the community approach to the care of the elderly which has been emphasised earlier in this chapter. One proviso in Slattery and Bourne's thesis is that 50 per cent of the geriatric beds will be acute, a figure higher than that proposed by the current thinking of the Department of Health and Social Security.

Psychogeriatric Services

In parallel with the geriatric medical service must be a psychiatric service. It is well recognised that the elderly suffer from mental illness and mental infirmity. The incidence of mental illness amongst the elderly population is considerable and a recent survey suggested an incidence of about 30 per cent for depression but the incidence of moderate to severe depression needing active treatment is probably about 15 per cent, about half of whom may require either treatment or advice with regard to treatment from a hospital-based service. The incidence of dementia is less, in the order of 6 per cent. However, it increases with age being 13 per cent of those over 75 years and 22 per cent of those over 80 years. Consequently the need for psychiatric treatment among the elderly is considerable. The resources needed to meet this need are similar to those required by the geriatric medical service. The clinical and day place requirements are shown in Table 2.2. In addition the psychogeriatric team has a considerable community role in the management and treatment of mental illness and mental infirmity. In most services the psychiatrists are supported by community nursing teams and the operational policy necessary to provide an efficient service is described in Chapter 10.

Demographic and Epidemiological Aspects

The resources necessary to meet the needs of the elderly will obviously depend on the number of elderly in the area under consideration and the age and social structure of that population. The younger the overall age of the elderly population the more active they are likely to be and the less help they will need. Similarly, the smaller the proportion of elderly in the population the smaller will be the requirement for resources. An area that has a population containing only 10 per cent elderly (over 65 years) will obviously need less in the way of services and resources than an area with 30–40 per cent elderly, such as one might meet on the south coast of England. A population with a large proportion of the elderly over 75 years and over 85 years will need more resources since it is well known that morbidity and frailty increase with age. This is a problem which faces the UK as a whole. Population projections suggest that while the population aged 65–75 years will remain fairly constant at a little over 8 million, those over 75 years are expected to increase by more than one-third while those over 85 years may increase by more than a half from a little under ½ million to a little more than ¾ million. This will mean that the current resources for the elderly will be under a considerable strain and their efficient utilisation will be essential.

Apart from the population's age structure, its distribution in the area and its social structure are vitally important. Elderly who live in old housing in town centres will require more services than those who live in modern up-to-date housing. A population with a large number of social class 4 and 5 will similarly need more since this group are poorer and often have inferior housing. Other aspects to be considered are the proportion living alone and the proportion of families unwilling or unable to provide support for their elderly dependants. This may occur in areas which provide good work opportunities for women or areas with poor public transport facilities or where communications are difficult.

Surveys have suggested that about one-fifth to one-quarter of the elderly in a standard UK population are likely to need the services of geriatric medicine and in assessing likely needs this is a useful figure to bear in mind.

Manpower Needs

The resources necessary to provide a geriatric service have been discussed at some length but very little mention has been made of the manpower necessary, with the exception of home help and social workers (Table 2.1). The manpower requirements are considerable and some of the figures given in the Wessex Regional Hospital Board's Working Party Report of 1972 are given in Appendix B to this chapter. These, however, only relate to the hospital service and it should be remembered that the higher the turnover of patients the more staff that will be required.

Conclusion

Assessment of need is a complex and difficult matter. It would seem that the first step is to define what are reasonable needs having taken the characteristics of the area into consideration and then to assess what resources are available within the area to meet them. Deficiencies can then be defined and arrangements made to meet them either by reorganisation and better use of existing resources or by planning to provide new resources.

This poses the question as to what is 'reasonable' and this will have to be decided by taking into account the traditions and attitudes of the people living in the area. It must be remembered that 'wants' will always exceed 'needs', and 'needs' exceed 'resources'. This may be an advantage since a shortage of resources should mean that their use is better planned and that waste is diminished. Any service which sets out to meet the 'wants' of all will almost certainly be wastefully overprovided with resources.

Appendix A: A Checklist of the Needs and Requirements Within a Given Area

NEED	*REQUIREMENT*
1. Information *re* needs and rights	Information centre run by local authority or voluntary organisation. Appropriate literature distribution
2. Early detection and prevention of disease	Family medicine and community medicine geared to this need. Age/sex register available. Education of family medicine staff. Appropriate family medicine record system
3. Receive medical treatment when physical and mental problems arise	Good family medicine organisation with integration of nurses, doctors and health visitors, and supported by ancillary services, viz. physiotherapy, occupational therapy, chiropody, aids, night nursing/attendant scheme, laundry service, bath attendants. Close links between hospital geriatric medical and psychiatric service; good community medicine and other supporting medical services such as audiology, ophthalmology and dental
4. Receive guidance with regard to social problems, isolation and loneliness	Good social services with social work, day centres, day clubs, holiday relief, good neighbour schemes, neighbourhood care, meals-on-wheels, lunch clubs, home help, aids schemes
5. Receive advice on retirement and how to continue to develop skills	Pre- and post-retirement education. Adult educational schemes. Links between young and old. Workshops for the elderly
6. Appropriate housing and residential accommodation	Schemes for altering existing housing when disability occurs. Suitable housing for elderly including warden-supervised housing. Residential homes (local authority, voluntary and private)
7. To receive specialist care in hospital as necessary	In addition to acute medical and surgical specialties, geriatric medical and psychiatric services with beds, outpatient clinics and day hospital places. (Nursing home and private hospital places should be taken into consideration)

Appendix B: Medical Staffing

Basic allowance:

> 3½ sessions per week of medical staff of all grades including consultant, per 100 admissions per year (assumes turnover of 4 patients/bed, i.e. 35 sessions for a 250 bedded unit).

Additional allowances:

> 22 sessions per 50 day hospital places.
> 11 to 15 sessions to cover psychogeriatric inpatients and day patients (or in the case of psychiatrist to cover geriatric consultations).
> 7 to 11 sessions to cover liaison and consultations with other specialties, e.g. to cover joint ward rounds with acute departments, stroke unit, orthopaedic geriatric unit, other specialist use of beds, local authority and voluntary agencies.
> 0-44 sessions (average 22 sessions) to cover factors such as outpatients, domiciliary assessment visiting, teaching, research, geographical scatter, a higher proportion of over 75s in the population, etc.

Grades of Medical Staff

E.g. staff for 250 beds:

Consultant	2 consultants
Senior registrar/registrar	2 registrars
House physicians	at least 2 (including SHO grade)
GP clinical assistant	General practitioners may be usefully employed in community hospitals

Nursing Staff and Paramedical Staff

Nurses	Minimum of 1:1.25 all beds.
	1:6 day hospital places (These will need adjustment to fit negotiated working hours, e.g. 37½ hours/week)
Social workers	2:250 beds of all types
	1:50 day hospital places
Social work clerks	2:250 beds of all types
Physiotherapists	4:250 beds of all types
	2:30 day hospital places (maximum of 3)
	1:250 psychogeriatric beds of all types
Occupational therapists	4:250 beds of all types
	2:30 day hospital places (max. of 3)
Therapy aides	12:250 beds of all types
	4:30 day hospital places

Secretarial and Administrative Staff

Secretary to department (higher clerical officer)	1:250 beds of all types
Secretary to consultant (personal secretary)	1:250 beds of all types
Clerk/shorthand typist	1:250 beds of all types
	1:30 day hospital places

References

Akhtar, A.J., Broe, G.A., Crombie, A., McLean, W.M.R., Andrews, G.R. and Caird, F.I. (1973). 'Disability and dependence in the elderly at home'. *Age and Ageing*, 2, 102

Anderson, F. (1978). 'The early detection and prevention of disease in the elderly', in *Recent Advances in Geriatric Medicine*, Vol. 1, B. Isaacs (ed.). Churchill Livingstone, Edinburgh

Anderson, W.F. and Cowan, N.R. (1955). 'A consultative health centre for older people'. *Lancet*, ii, 239

Andrews, G.R., Cowan, N.R. and Anderson, W.F. (1971). 'The practice of geriatric medicine in the community, an evaluation of the place of health centres', in *Problems and Progress in Medical Care, Essays on Current Research*, 5th series. G. McLachlan (ed.). Oxford University Press

Beverfelt, E. (1980). 'Norway', in *International Handbook on Ageing: Contemporary Developments and Research*. E. Palmore (ed.). Macmillan, London

Butler, R.N. (1969). 'Age-ism another form of bigotry.' *The Gerontologist*, 9, 243

Bytheway, W.R. (1980). 'United Kingdom,' in *International Handbook on Ageing: Contemporary Developments and Research*. E. Palmore (ed.). Macmillan, London

Coleman, P.G. (1975). 'Social Gerontology in the Netherlands.' *The Gerontologist*, 15, 3, 257

DeLargy, J. (1957). 'Six weeks in: Six weeks out.' *Lancet*, i. 418

DHSS (1979). *Nutrition and health in old age*, RHFS16. HMSO, London

Dodd, K., Clarke, M. and Palmer, R.L. (1980). 'Misplacement of the elderly in hospitals and residential homes: A survey and follow up.' *Health Trends*, 12, 74

Dumazedier, J. (1972). 'Cultural mutations in post industrial societies.' Proceedings of 3rd International Course of Social Gerontology

Hall, M.R.P. (1980). 'Supplying the demand.' *Health and Social Service Journal*, 17 Oct., 1347

Hall, M.R.P., MacLennan, W.J. and Lye, M.D.W. (1978). *Medical Care of the Elderly*. HM + M publishers, Aylesbury; Springer Publishing Company, New York

Irvine, R.E. (1980). 'Geriatric day hospitals: Present trends.' *Health Trends*, 12, 68

MacLennan, W.J. and Hall, M.R.P. (1980). 'Geriatric clinics in general practitioner surgeries'. *Practitioner*, 224, 687

Munday, M. and Rowe, J. (1979). 'Care of the elderly in Devon. A project funded by the King's Fund to assess the needs of the elderly in GP practices'

Opit, L.J. (1977). 'Domiciliary care for the elderly sick: Economy or neglect'. *British Medical Journal*, 1, 30

Parnell, J.W. and Naylor, R. (1973). *Home for the weekend – Back on Monday*. Queen's Institute of District Nursing publication, London

Robertson, J.C. and Haines, J.R. (1977). 'A community/hospital home aids loan scheme.' *Salisbury Medical Bulletin*, 30, 143

Ruikka, I. (1971). 'Geriatrics in Finland.' *World Medicine Journal*, 18, 49

Schwenger, C.W. (1971). 'Sociomedical care of the aged.' *World Medicine Journal*, 18, 42

Slattery, M. and Bourne, A. (1979). 'Norms and recent trends in geriatrics.' *J. Clinical Experimental Gerontology*, 1(1), 79

Spackman, A. (1980). Personal communication

Townsend, P. (1962). *The last refuge. A survey of residential institutions and homes for the aged in England and Wales.* Routledge and Kegan Paul, London

Wager, R. (1972). *Care of the elderly – an exercise in cost benefit analysis.* Institute of Municipal Treasurers and Accountants, London

Williamson, J. (1966). 'Ageing in modern society.' Paper presented to the Royal Society of Health, Edinburgh, 9 November

Williamson, J., Lowther, C.P. and Gray, S. (1966). 'The use of Health Visitors in preventive geriatrics.' *Gerontologia Clinica*, 8, 362

Zonneveld, R.J. van (1980). 'The Netherlands', in *International Handbook on Ageing: Contemporary Developments and Research*. E. Palmore (ed.). Macmillan, London

3 OPERATIONAL POLICIES

J. Pathy

It is recognised that geriatric medicine is a relatively new area of medical practice. It has been regarded by many as an administrative necessity rather than as a clinical discipline. It suffers from the legacy of the Poor Law and the era of the chronic irremediable sick storehouse concept. The term 'geriatrics' has different connotations to different people, but it is popularly regarded as a field of health care which acts as a repository for demented, physically disabled and socially unacceptable old people. The tragic restraints, barriers and hurdles that have often to be overcome are mainly due to emotional misconceptions and, in no small measure, to culpable ignorance.

A keen observer visiting departments of geriatric medicine in the United Kingdom will be struck both by a theme that is common to a majority of units and by major policy differences. Inherited hospital and community resources and geographical considerations may influence operational policies. It is clear that the major determinant influencing fundamental objectives in the past has been the philosophy of the physician responsible for the development of the geriatric service.

'Operational Policy' may be defined as a statement of the aims, methods and processes of an organisation.

Achievement of an Overall Policy

Precisely defined objectives based on informed data form the cornerstone of appropriate operational policies for a developing department. The aims by which ultimate objectives are achieved require adequate exposition. The commonest basis for failure is insensitive haste and inadequate communication. If policies are not to be built on sand, considerable spadework is necessary to form a sound foundation on which the superstructure is to be slowly built. Explanation, discussion, widespread teaching to many disciplines and the utmost sensitivity to contrary views, often held with fervour and deep conviction, are some of the essential building implements.

Operational policies are designed to achieve a set of defined objectives. In the development or recasting of a department of geriatric medicine, it should be appreciated that a stated goal may have to be reached in stages. This will require a set of operational strategies to reach each intermediate phase. Operational policies should be sufficiently flexible to respond to the changing patterns of society and of medicine.

General 'Area' Operational Policies

It is mandatory to establish a comprehensive data base relevant to the total resources and facilities in the functional geographical area in which a new or revamped department of geriatric medicine is to develop. Critical data components would include the operational policies of other clinical, diagnostic and administrative departments, nursing policies, local fiscal policies, statutory community policies and resources, the additional resources of the voluntary and private sectors and policies which influence their availability. Ambulance resources and general transport policies may be crucial to the speed and direction in which a geriatric service can develop.

Historically geriatric medicine rose from a system of custodial care – a system based on a philosophy that illness and disability in old age was generally incurable and therefore untreatable. The consequence of this tenet was that of permanent care in institutions far removed from those areas of medicine where diagnosis and treatment were practised. An awakening of public conscience led to the dawn of well meaning and largely misplaced sentimentalism which changed plain walls and bare windows for colour and chintz curtains. This was heralded as an era of enlightenment by many. Few will deny the dramatic advances that have been achieved in the United Kingdom in the medicine of old age in little more than 25 years. Nevertheless it is clear that the spectrum of medical services provided by different units varies from little more than an hotel and custodial caring service to the comprehensive provision of specialised general medical services for the elderly sick and disabled. It is probable that no department of geriatric medicine under the supervision of a specialist in this discipline in the UK practises a wholly custodial care function. Many departments only take 'cold' referrals from general specialties after the acute phase of an illness has subsided and physical disability or difficulty in resettlement back into the community appear as barriers to discharge from hospital. The expertise offered by the specialist in geriatric medicine in this situation is the provision of an active rehabilitation service and the administrative ability to harness the relevant community resources, both statutory and voluntary, to facilitate return to the patient's household or to a sheltered form of care.

At the other end of the spectrum are departments which provide an extensive range of diagnostic and therapeutic resources to either the majority or to all 'medical' patients above a defined age, i.e. a policy of regarding geriatric medicine as an age-defined specialty. Within these significant variations in the practice of geriatric medicine in the United Kingdom and Ireland, three broad operational concepts can be identified.

(1) The practice of a limited role in the totality of geriatric medicine where no acutely ill patients are directly admitted.
(2) Acceptance of a small proportion of acutely ill patients whose medical conditions fall within proscribed limits.
(3) Provision of a broad area of expertise in disease of later life with the admission of all or the majority of medically ill old people irrespective of the acuteness of the disease(s).

It is apposite to consider each of these broad variants and to discuss some of the general operational policies subserving them.

Departments that Exclude Direct Admission of the Acutely Ill Elderly

The specialised expertise that these departments provide is primarily in the field of physical rehabilitation and social resettlement. It was these two areas of expertise that the late Marjorie Warren (see Chapter 1) pioneered with such distinction and success. It requires comment that many of the patients with whom she achieved such notable success were significantly younger than the average patient entering departments of geriatric medicine today. (This is based on personal experience of many visits to her department in the second half of the 1950s.) The level of organisation of the rehabilitation services, though often restricted in available personnel, tends to be excellent. In practice many of these departments devote 50-70 per cent of the total departmental beds to a continuing-care service. Long waiting lists due to slow throughput often result in unnecessary or irremediable deformity or lessened patient morale. The requirement of medical staff is lower, but the breadth of training is circumscribed. Burley *et al.* (1979) have shown that the average duration of stay of elderly patients in general medical wards can be appreciably shortened by introducing the skills of physicians in geriatric medicine early in the disability. The Hospital Inpatient Enquiry for England and Wales (Preliminary tables, HMSO, 1978) showed that bed use factor (i.e. approximately the number of patients passing through one bed per year) in general medicine was 30, but in geriatric medicine only 4.8. The unit cost per occupied bed in low-turnover units is considerably less than the higher turnover units, but the cost per patient is often astronomical. Adams (1964) has highlighted the danger of a department of geriatric medicine taking on the role of a clinical undertaker.

Departments Admitting a Proportion of Elderly Persons with Proscribed Acute Conditions

This arrangement may be conceptual or due to a lack of general hospital facilities to the department of geriatric medicine. Absence of surgical facilities may necessitate exclusion of patients with gastrointestinal bleeding. Resources may be so limited that all serious medical emergencies must be refused. A review of historical policies will often indicate the acceptance of additional beds in unwanted peripheral hospitals as an expedient to reduce waiting lists. These policies ultimately prove shortsighted. Available evidence indicates that few high-cost beds, i.e. beds in district general hospitals, provide a more appropriate and effective service to the elderly community. However, bed turnover is only one criterion of the level of service. Isaacs *et al.* (1972) have pleaded for the appropriate provision for the 'hard-core' patients. Certain units have the requisite resources, but have an operational policy which excludes the seriously ill. It must be questionable whether this policy is legitimate on economic grounds, if on no other.

Departments Admitting All or Most Medical Emergencies Above a Specified Age Limit

Where this policy is operational, it is mandatory that a significant proportion of the departmental beds are sited within a district general hospital with the immediate availability of other major disciplines and equal access to appropriate diagnostic, therapeutic and outpatient facilities. Medical and nursing staff levels can be no less than for equivalent general medical departments. Departments of geriatric medicine which are recognised for specialist training in this discipline have doctors whose background has to include adequate experience in general medicine and who have to hold a postgraduate degree in general medicine. Their training is in all aspects of the medicine of old age and distinction between acute or chronic illness is irrelevant. A policy of postgraduate training of medical, nursing and paramedical staff as an on-going function is of great importance.

The specialist in geriatric medicine may require the expertise of the neurologist, dermatologist or other specialist as do his colleagues in general medicine. The strength of an age-related policy lies in the opportunity to introduce a problem-orientated and holistic approach to the elderly at whatever stage disease may present itself. Most chronic disorders commence as acute conditions. The protagonists of an age-defined admission policy maintain that the basic general management approach to the elderly acutely ill or the more chronically ill are conceptually similar. The acute event may disguise other significant disorders which, though possibly irrelevant to the acute condition, may cumulatively impair an attainable level of independence and quality of life. Delays incurred by a predominantly secondary transfer policy reduce the success rate of rehabilitation; difficulty in discharging patients is proportional to the duration of hospitalisation.

Where an age-defined admission policy is adopted, varying age limits are used, primarily on the basis that with a given allocation of resources, it is only possible to cope with all patients over 75 and a limited proportion of patients aged 65-74 (Bagnell *et al.*, 1977; Evans *et al.*, 1971) or all patients over 70 (Das Gupta, 1980). O'Brien *et al.* (1973) found that they were able to cope with all medical admissions aged 65 and over. The Department of Geriatric Medicine in South Glamorgan offers an age-related admission policy for all medical patients aged 65 and over. The right of the family doctor to seek the physician or department that he believes will provide the optimum service for his patient is considered paramount. Figure 3.1 shows all admissions over the age of 65 to general medical and geriatric medical beds in South Glamorgan (all inter-unit transfers and intermittent admissions are excluded from the figures for admissions to the geriatric unit). It is relevant to indicate that both in general medicine and in geriatric medicine, male emergencies predominate in the age group of 65-70.

Table 3.1 lists those high-turnover units which give data for available beds, population aged 65 and over (1971 census) and deaths and discharges per year.

The review by Hodkinson and Jeffreys (1972) cannot be included in Table 3.1 as their data only related to beds in Northwick Park Hospital

Figure 3.1: Admissions in General Medicine and Geriatric Medicine—65 Years and Over Via the Emergency Bed Bureau South Glamorgan Health Authority (T), (1978)

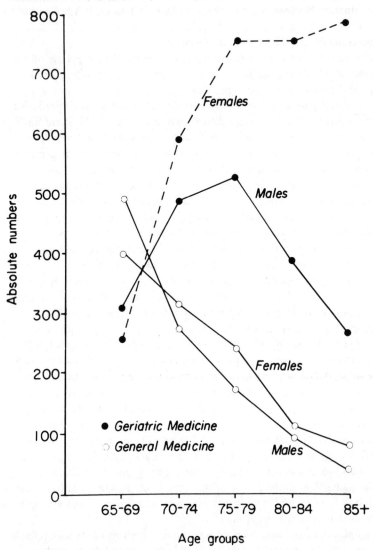

(Middlesex) and not to the total available beds. The bed use factor was not recorded by all authors and it has therefore been calculated in these instances. It is evident that these departments have a higher bed use

Table 3.1: Data from High-turnover Geriatric Units

Authors	Beds	Population 65 and over	Discharges	Bed use factor
O'Brien *et al.*	296	32,925	2,041	7
Bagnell *et al.*	433	53,585	4,294	9
Das Gupta	169	18,560	1,593	9
Sth. Glamorgan H. A. (T) (1978)	430	56,000	5,345	11.9

factor than the mean for England and Wales. Hodkinson and Jeffreys (1972) were unable to show that high admission rates reflected increased availability of beds. On the contrary many slow-turnover departments have a larger allocation of beds. The one factor common to all these high-turnover departments is the availability of a major proportion of the total beds in district general hospitals.

Operational Factors Pertinent to High-turnover Units: Waiting Lists

The presence of a waiting list is 'more a matter of choice of its medical staff than a reflection of local circumstances' (Hodkinson and Jeffreys, 1972). High-turnover units tend to have no waiting lists, low-turnover units almost consistently have a considerable waiting list. A waiting list is an anathema in geriatric practice. Time is rarely on the side of the elderly. A 24-hour hospital service is essential, prompt hospital admission generally allows the optimum opportunity for effective management and early return to the community. Crises admissions due to waiting lists not only lessen the effectiveness of medical management, but effectively destroy the trust of the family doctor, relatives and the community at large in the reliability of a department of geriatric medicine to supply an essential hospital resource at an appropriate point in time.

The Function of Hospital Beds in Departments of Geriatric Medicine

Two differing policies have been adopted in the United Kingdom. Infrequently no distinction is made as to whether patients require short-term diagnostic and therapeutic facilities, predominant

Figure 3.2: The Function of Hospital Beds in Departments of Geriatric Medicine: Two Different Policies (a and b)

(a)

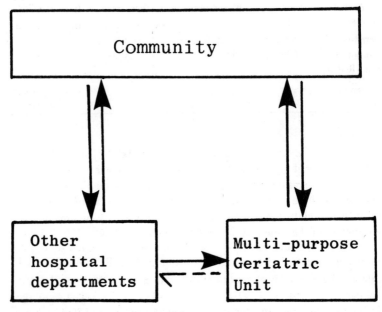

(b)

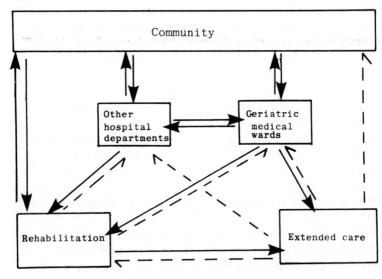

rehabilitation facilities or extended or continuing-care services. (Bagnell *et al.*, 1977) (Figure 3.2a). The advantages claimed for this policy are: higher nurse and patient morale; continuity of care by the same team of medical, nursing and remedial staff; and a reduction in the overall numbers of continuing-care beds. Our past experience of multi-purpose wards indicates a significant reluctance on the part of some relatives to agree to appropriate hospital discharge on the basis that nearby patients have been allowed to remain indefinitely. District general hospitals are considerably more expensive than extended-care hospitals. In many areas it is only possible for patients requiring extended (or continuing) care to be near to relatives or friends by utilising small local units.

The alternative policy uses beds according to the diagnostic, therapeutic or functional needs of the patient (Figure 3.2b). Particular wards or hospitals may serve identifiable roles and terms such as acute assessment wards, rehabilitation wards and long-stay wards are in common use. The terms associated with these functional areas are unfortunate and often misleading. It is difficult to find acceptable alternatives, but 'geriatric medical beds' most closely describes the role of so-called assessment beds. 'Extended care' is more positive and often more appropriate than long stay or continuing care. Rehabilitation is a phase in the overall management of most ill elderly persons. However, we believe that those patients who have recovered from the acute phase of their condition, e.g. a limb amputation or a stroke, but require a major rehabilitation programme over a few to several weeks, progress most expeditiously in wards specially geared and equipped for this aspect of management. As in busy general medical wards, this group of patients is often subconsciously given a lesser degree of available staff time when they are in competition with heavy intakes of elderly medical emergencies. If the organisational policy is carefully designed, the system of functional separation, with general hospital siting for all 'active treatment' beds, is compatible with high turnover and a wide spectrum service requiring only minimal extended-care beds.

Unfortunately many departments with hospital facilities based on the 'traditional' functional division are overendowed with continuing-care beds and often have few or no beds in district general hospitals. The majority of elderly patients for whom hospital admission is justified have complex problems and often multi-system disease requiring a high degree of clinical and diagnostic acumen and not infrequently sophisticated resources. It is facile to believe that optimum restorative success will be achieved in the absence of those facilities which are essential to obtain appropriate levels of success in other age groups. A policy directed towards trading diagnostic and therapeutic facilities for an increase in continuing-care beds is a policy of pawning the birthright of the elderly sick without a hope of redemption at the end of the day. An operational policy may, with advantage, state that no patient is admitted to the department of geriatric medicine except for the expressed purpose of diagnosis and treatment directed towards resettlement of all patients back in the community. Failures to meet this objective will of necessity occur, but are likely to be greater if the policy is less positively assertive.

Domiciliary Assessment of Non-emergency Referrals for Hospital Admission

This was an almost universal practice during the inception phase of geriatric medicine in the United Kingdom. Information based on the replies received from 101 departments of geriatric medicine in 1972 (Pathy *et al.*, 1972), indicated that all but three departments carried out a pre-admission assessment of non-emergency cases by a hospital-based doctor in a varying proportion of cases (Figure 3.3).
Pre-admission assessments by hospital medical staff permits an appraisal of the social background against which the patient's medical condition can be evaluated and future management planned. It also helps to decide the level of priority on a waiting list for hospital admission. Pathy and his colleagues (1972) reported their experience since 1961 of pre-admission assessment of selected requests for non-emergency admissions by full-time health visitors specialising in geriatric medicine. This study indicated that pre-admission assessment by a doctor showed little objective benefit over an assessment provided by an adequately trained health visitor. The proportion of medical time consumed in undertaking pre-admission assessment visits must be related to the time required to care for those patients in hospital. Many medical assessments are more profitably undertaken in an outpatient clinic with social and domestic data provided where necessary by a skilled health visitor or social worker. Where a geriatric service is newly introduced into an area, pre-admission assessment of non-emergency patients by a consultant during the formative months has considerable value in providing appraisal of the social structure of an area and an overview of the medical practice of the various primary physicians.

Figure 3.3: Histogram Showing Percentages of Non-emergency Referrals Assessed by Medical Staff of Units Before Admission in 101 Geriatric Departments in England and Wales

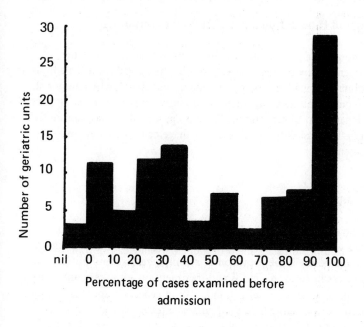

Multidisciplinary Ward Rounds – Multidisciplinary Case Conferences

Few would deny that the multidisciplinary approach to patient management is the hallmark of geriatric medicine. Numerous variations on multidisciplinary ward rounds are practised in different departments. All have the advantage that the members of the team see the patient together and are aware of his range of problems, his progress and future management plans. Each member of the team is continuously learning from the expertise of the others. This type of ward round is time-consuming, though effective. A multidisciplinary round may be organised subsequent to a 'medical' round with greater emphasis on particular patients. Case conferences have the advantage of being held away from the immediate vicinity of the patient and economise on time, but suffer from the lack of visual appreciation of a patient's progress. Wright and Lubbock (1979) have tried to overcome this disadvantage with considerable success by showing weekly videotapes of patient progress to the relevant health care staff. However, no case conference or videotape can convey the nuances of the mental and physical change that can be witnessed on a multidisciplinary ward round.

Transfer of Patients from General Medical Departments

This should rarely be required in high-turnover units. Following assessment, many of these patients can be discharged from the admitting discipline with guidance on general management and, where required, advice on organising appropriate community support services. If transfer to a department of geriatric medicine is appropriate, delay substantially reduces the possibility of successful management and community re-settlement.

Day Hospitals

This subject is discussed in detail in Chapter 4. However, day hospital policies will influence the overall operational policy of a department. Where the policy is the provision of a comprehensive multidisciplinary hospital resource for diagnosis and treatment on a non-residential basis, the siting of a day hospital within a district general hospital is the only meaningful decision. Where the policy is directed to simple rehabilitative or essentially caring roles, the siting of a day hospital is less restrictive, but the demands on inpatient service are magnified.

Day Centres

Day centres serve a critical supporting function to day hospitals. A proportion of patients requiring day hospital therapeutic resources will profit considerably from the incidental supportive role. This is seen particularly in the socially vulnerable. Once the need for day hospital resources has been met, a supportive day centre provision may serve to enable the elderly person to be maintained in the community. It was our early experience that where no day centres exist, encouragement of local authorities and voluntary organisations to develop these facilities was an appropriate policy for the vulnerable elderly and it ensured the continued functioning of the day hospital system.

Outpatient Clinics

As with other disciplines, the appropriate siting is a district general
hospital. Any deviation from this policy will limit appropriate diagnostic
and other disciplinary facilities or may entail the use of inappropriate
resources, e.g. hospital admission. Once a department establishes a
comprehensive range of hospital resources it can broaden its policy to
undertake outpatient clinics for selected patients in health centres and
small peripheral hospitals, particularly in predominantly rural areas.
This has considerable advantages for patients, hospital staff and family
doctors. Geriatric medical outpatient clinics sited in family doctor health
clinics often draw on a different clientele than hospital-based clinics.
The early manifestation of disease or symptom complexes are more
likely to be seen in these clinics and afford a precious opportunity for
mutual education and an appropriate situation to teach the value of
early total assessment of the health-impaired patient.

The range of services and the emphasis on individual services must of
necessity vary from one department of geriatric medicine to another,
depending on local requirements, resources and policies. Caution is
essential to ensure that apparent lack of resources does not become an
alibi for failure to pursue policies which are manifestly beneficial for
the elderly community. Determination, fortitude and repeated exposition,
both verbal and written, supported by essential data, will normally permit
most logical policies to evolve gradually. Evolution rather than revolution
is perhaps a useful guiding principle. The overall range of services
provided by departments of geriatric medicine in the UK is extensive
and many are mentioned in other chapters. However, it is essential to
appreciate that the development of each one of them will depend on an
overt policy decision. The nature of each service is consequential on
agreed operational policies. It would appear germane to the brief of
this chapter to illustrate some of the commonly recognised service
provisions.

Intermittent Admissions

De Largy's 'Six weeks in: Six weeks out' (De Largy, 1957) scheme of
relief for families caring for heavily disabled old people had the merit
of simplicity, but lacked the flexibility that is required to tailor a
hospital support scheme to the needs of an individual patient and his

major carers. If a department is to provide the minimum number of extended-care beds, which we believe to be the only sustainable policy in the face of an increasing demand of an ever ageing and more socially sophisticated society, some form of shared care is required for those for whom a hospital provision is appropriate. Whether this 'hospital resource' should be provided by the geriatric service, a general practitioner community hospital or by a private or voluntary nursing home, will depend on local policies and the availability of various alternative provisions. The majority of the available population will support the severely disabled elderly in the community if periodic relief is available prior to a point of irretrievable crisis.

Holiday Admissions

A policy which provides annual holiday relief to relatives or neighbours providing major support to heavily dependent old people has appeared to us to be critical. The provision of one or two weeks or, occasionally, longer periods of hospital admission has functioned successfully in South Glamorgan for 20 years. A domiciliary assessment is undertaken on all new referrals and this has resulted in approximately 30 per cent of all referrals being accommodated by other agencies. In our experience, where hospital admission is appropriate, a therapeutically orientated policy — usually physical therapy — has had merit and provides a positive health resource input during the brief inpatient stay.

Mental Disorders in the Elderly: Psychogeriatric Service

In a community survey, Kay *et al.* (1964) showed that 10 per cent of persons over 65 had evidence of chronic brain failure and Pasker *et al.* (1976) noted psychiatric problems in one-third of persons aged 65 and over who were receiving nursing care (at home, in residential care or in hospital). The Department of Health and Social Security has produced guidelines (1972) to indicate respective areas of responsibility between psychiatrists and physicians in geriatric medicine in relation to old persons suffering from mental health problems. The division of responsibility between these two disciplines is to an extent arbitary as the elderly tend to have mental and physical phenomena closely intertwined. Patients with acute confusional states or predominant physical disease are regarded as the responsibility of physicians in geriatric medicine and predominant psychotic or established organic confusional or dementing disorders are considered more appropriately managed by the psychiatric services. Arie (1971) is broadly in agreement with this concept, but Enoch and Howells (1971) believe that organic mental disorders in the elderly are not the responsibility of psychiatrists. In the face of opposing opinions, local operational policies will depend on positive dialogue. Nevertheless the availability of adequate resources in both disciplines has a major impact on policy decisions.

Psychogeriatric Assessment Units

The establishment of such units was a major component of DHSS policy (1970, 1972). The establishment of effective psychogeriatric assessment units requires close functional interrelationship between consultants both in psychiatry and geriatric medicine and the social services departments (see Chapter 10). Clearly defined admission, discharge or transfer policies are the *sine qua non* for success. Too often deficiencies exist in one or more components and ultimately the assessment unit takes on a continuing care role. Arie and Dunn (1973) showed that it was possible to provide an effective combined assessment service utilising only a four-bed unit for an over-65 population of 25,000.

Joint Orthopaedic – Geriatric Medical Units

An increasing awareness of the positive value of joint orthopaedic-geriatric medical wards or units has become apparent in recent years, (Devas and Irvine, 1963 and 1969). Our own experience since 1963 also confirms the effective contribution of geriatric medicine to the medical, rehabilitative and social resettlement functions of these combined wards. Our more recent experience of the provision of early geriatric medical intervention services indicates that the policy of early pre- and post-operative collaborative involvement considerably improves the overall management of the older traumatic orthopaedic patient (Chapter 11).

The Lower Limb Amputee

The elderly amputee often affords a model upon which good geriatric medical practice should be based. The technical operative procedure is outside the competence of the physician, though the exact technique significantly concerns him in relation to subsequent rehabilitation and acceptable prosthetic management. The patient has to face a major, psychologically-traumatic procedure; he will experience an acute post-operative catabolic state and will require a planned programme of rehabilitation and social resettlement. Our experience is that the provision of this service within the ambit of a department of geriatric medicine has led to excellent reciprocal general and vascular surgical facilities. It is self-evident that an operational policy that aims to provide a rehabilitation service for considerable numbers of elderly lower limb amputees will be influenced by available resources.

Urology

This is only separated from many other essential areas of surgery in that it represents, *par excellence*, a service where collaborative arrangements can provide the elderly with excellent overall management in a manner which is mutually beneficial to both urological and geriatric medical departments.

Stroke Units

The incidence of stroke disease rises precipitously over the age of 65 and particularly after 75. Isaacs *et al.* (1976) found that one-third of patients referred to a stroke unit in Glasgow were under 65, 40 per cent in the decade 65-74, and one-third were aged 75 and over. Kennedy (1976) considered that stroke units were most appropriately located within a department of geriatric medicine. Garroway *et al.* (1980 a & b) found that stroke patients initially improved to a greater extent when treated in a stroke unit within the geriatric service than when treated in district general hospitals, but the benefit at the end of one year was the same in both groups. Possibly the greater earlier improvement could have been maintained if patients and relatives had counselling following hospital discharge. Pathy (1974) showed that 70 per cent of stroke patients who survived for at least three months were able to continue reasonably independent lives and that continued counselling and the participation of spouse, relatives or caring friends in the later stages of rehabilitation have proved a valuable policy and prevented regression. It has been our policy to provide a rehabilitation unit dealing mainly with strokes and amputees, rather than with a single disease entity. The operational policy relating to the rehabilitation of strokes will depend on local facilities and patient requirements, and on the attitudes of physicians and rehabilitation therapists. There is serious need for scientifically controlled studies before operational policies can reflect facts rather than impressions.

Counselling

Counselling services for relatives and patients are patchy and cover differing areas of need. Counselling of patients, relatives or friends is particularly crucial where residual, physical, mental or communication problems are present. Recent counselling clinics for elderly patients discharged from hospital following a myocardial infarction have been invaluable (Pathy and Peach, 1980). The possible introduction of counselling schemes requires a regular reappraisal of total departmental resources to ensure that a degree of fragmentation does not occur that spreads too many services too thinly for overall efficiency and effectiveness.

Social Services Departments

Following the implementation of the Seebohm Report (1968) in 1974, the dichotomy between health and social services was extended. The provision of an integrated geriatric service was potentially eliminated. In practice, mutually agreed local arrangements allow circumvention of many restrictive barriers. It is critical to negotiate a formula which allows the siting in departments of geriatric medicine of medical social workers whose full-time commitment is to the elderly. It is our experience that a policy in which patients and available relatives are seen by a social worker within 24 hours of hospital admission permits a realistic assessment of the patients' social background and engenders a positive attitude to subsequent domestic resettlement in both patient and relative. This also provides reasonable time for the mobilisation of statutory and voluntary support resources should they be required. Wilson and Wilson (1971) record that 98 per cent of elderly inpatients need one or more social services, particularly home nursing.

Social Services Residential Accommodation

Where no hospital waiting list exists, the policy effecting hospital admission of residents of local authority residential homes should in no way differ essentially from that relating to older persons in their own homes. Where a hospital inpatient cannot personally cope or be supported in the community even with statutory and voluntary services, local authority residential care may have to be considered. It is our view that this option is accepted too readily, but if it is appropriate, many areas operate an exchange system, i.e. agree to accept a very dependent ex-local authority resident to achieve a vacancy for the transfer of an inpatient. Braverman and Baldock (1980) discuss the policy of a defined number of places in local authority residential homes being specifically set apart for the use of a department of geriatric medicine. This scheme has considerable merit, but requires consistent discipline to avoid unnecessary utilisation of a less appropriate resource due to administrative convenience.

The foregoing discussion has primarily revolved around strategic and conceptual operational policies aimed at providing a predetermined range of services to the elderly sick. However, a wide spectrum of day-to-day operational policies require to be formulated to achieve a harmoniously functioning department that is based on a clearly defined and accepted internal administrative structure.

A policy of medical assessment of current or prospective residents of local authority homes for the elderly significantly reduces misplacement and unnecessary dependency. Policies directed towards this area of practice require co-operation and collaboration with family doctors and social services departments. While the utmost scrutiny is required to prevent undue stretching of scarce resources, it is clear that a geriatric medical service cannot confine its activities entirely to a hospital-based and orientated function and escape unscathed in the final analysis.

Discussion of a comprehensive catalogue of the multitude of minor policies dictated by local needs or idiosyncrasies has no virtue. Most departments of geriatric medicine in the United Kingdom initially appointed a single consultant to develop a service. The direction of that development was influenced by the philosophy of the individual consultant who had to devote considerable administrative endeavours to implement change. With an increasing number of consultants in a department, potential disharmony and contention may occur if the original consultant remains personally responsible for all decision-making. It is imperative that there is flexibility that both permits and actively

encourages new concepts. Sterility and slow fossilisation will character-
ise any branch of medicine that regards the introduction of new areas
of expertise as a threat to an established system. Change merely for the
sake of change equally has no merit.

No department can function effectively and have the hallmark of
direction, unless its fundamental operational policies are consistent and
identifiable. Analysis and identification of the functional and administrative activities of a multi-consultant geriatric service are essential if
each consultant is to engage in a challenging and meaningful area of the
agreed policy structure of a department. It has proved helpful in some
large departments to operate a multidisciplinary committee of senior
medical and other senior health care staff with the chairman and
secretary drawn from the consultants in geriatric medicine, and each
serving a defined period of office. Day-to-day decision-making might be
undertaken by the consultant chairman, or in some departments by the
most senior colleague, if general consensus suggests that this is most
propitious.

Central Co-ordinating Office

The majority of departments have found it essential to develop a
central office for the reception of patient referrals and enquiries from a
wide range of agencies, e.g. general practitioners, other hospital services,
social services and health visitors. The organisation of intermittent and
holiday admissions and inter-unit transfers is readily undertaken
through this facility. The function of a 'central office' is not to duplicate
the role of medical records and hospital appointments departments.
These latter departments are not attuned to process many of the
enquiries and referrals in a form appropriate to the functioning of
departments of geriatric medicine. Many departments have beds, clinics
and day hospital services on several sites. The immediate access to a
central information system is invaluable. Computer storage and
retrieval of information decreases the delay in data availability. The
chances of communication gaps are greatly reduced if the offices of the
health visitors and social workers are situated near the central office.
Our experience over 10 years is that the appointment of an administrative
officer (Manager) significantly reduces the hiccups that tend to occur in
the administrative component of a department of geriatric medicine.

A department of geriatric medicine has a highly complex structure
and may be likened to an intricate machine. A machine is designed to

serve a function or set of functions. Each component has a definable role. The most efficient machine may be used ineffectively. The consultant in geriatric medicine has an architectural, administrative and managerial role in ensuring that a department is designed to fulfil defined objectives. The operational policies form the blueprint of the department. The blueprint must be capable of producing the desired working model.

References

Adams, G.F. (1964). 'Clinical Undertaking'. *Lancet*, i, 1055

Arie, T. (1971). 'Morale and the planning of psycho-geriatric services'. *British Medical Journal*, iii, 166

Arie, T. and Dunn, T. (1973). 'A "do-it-yourself" psycho-geriatric joint patient unit'. *Lancet*. ii, 1313

Bagnell, W.E., Datta, S.R., Knox, J. and Horrocks, P. (1977). 'Geriatric Medicine in Hull: A comprehensive service'. *British Medical Journal*, iii, 102

Braverman, A. and Baldock, P. (1980). 'An end to the old people's swop shop'. *Social Work Today*, 11, 45, 16

Burley, L.E., Currie, C.T., Smith, R.G. and Williamson, J. (1979). 'Contribution from geriatric medicine within acute medical wards'. *British Medical Journal*, 11, 90

Das Gupta, P.K. (1980). 'Developing an active geriatric service in Scunthorpe'. *Public Health London*, 94, 155

De Largy, J. (1957). 'Six weeks in: Six weeks out'. *Lancet*, i. 418

Department of Health and Social Security (1970). *Psychogeriatric assessment unit.* Circular H.M. (70) 11, DHSS, London

Department of Health and Social Security (1972). *Services for mental illness related to old age.* Circular H.M. (72) 71, DHSS, London

Devas, M.B. and Irvine, R.E. (1963). 'The geriatric orthopaedic unit'. *Journal of Bone and Joint Surgery*, 418, 630

Devas, M.B. and Irvine, R.E. (1969). 'The geriatric orthopaedic unit'. *British Journal of Geriatric Medicine*, 6, 19

Enoch, M.D. and Howells, J.D. (1971). *The organisation of psychogeriatrics.* Society of Clinical Psychiatrists (SCP), London

Evans, G.J., Hodkinson, H.M. and Mezey, A.G. (1971). 'The elderly sick – who looks after them?' *Lancet*, ii, 539

Garroway, W.M., Akhtar, A.J., Prescott, R.J. and Hockey, L. (1980a). 'Management of acute stroke in the elderly: preliminary results of a controlled trial'. *British Medical Journal*, 280, 1040

Garroway, W.M., Akhtar, A.J., Prescott, R.J. and Hockey, L. (1980b). 'Management of acute stroke in the elderly: follow-up of a controlled trial'. *British Medical Journal*, 281, 827

Hodkinson, H.M. and Jeffreys, P.M. (1972). 'Making hospital geriatrics work'. *British Medical Journal*, iv, 536

Hospital Inpatient Enquiry (preliminary tables). England and Wales (1978). HMSO

Isaacs, B., Livingston, M. and Neville, Y. (1972). *Survival of the Unfittest.* Routledge and Kegan Paul, London

Isaacs, N., Neville, T. and Rushford, I. (1976). 'The Stricken. The social consequence of a Stroke'. *Age and Ageing*, 5, 188

Kay, D.W.K., Beamish, P. and Roth, M. (1964). 'Old age mental disorders in Newcastle-upon-Tyne'. *British Journal of Psychiatry*, 110, 146

Kennedy, B.F. (1976). 'The Stroke Unit – a physiotherapist's views'. *Physiotherapy*, 62, 154

O'Brien, T.D., Joshie, D.M. and Warren, E.W. (1973). 'No apology for Geriatrics'. *British Medical Journal*, iv, 177

Pasker, D., Thomas, J.P. and Ashleigh, J.S. (1976). 'The elderly mentally ill – whose responsibility?' *British Medical Journal*, ii, 164

Pathy, M.S. (1974). 'Continuous combined assessment in rehabilitation of strokes'. *Gerontologia Clinica*, 17, 61

Pathy, M.S., Hughes, J.N.P. and White, W.M. (1972). 'The role of the Specialist Health Visitor in the Geriatric Team'. *Community Medicine*, 15, 206

Pathy, M.S. and Peach, H. (1980). 'Disability among the elderly after myocardial infarction. A 3-year follow-up'. *Journal of the Royal College of Physicians*, 14, 221

Seebohm Report (1968). *Report of the Committee on Local Authority and Allied Personal Social Services*. Cmnd. 3703, HMSO, London

Wilson, E.H. and Wilson, B.O. (1971). 'Integration of hospital and local authority services in the discharge of patients from a geriatric unit'. *Lancet*, ii, 864

Wollner, L. (1964). 'A joint appointment in Geriatrics'. *Gerontologia Clinica*, 2, 65

Wright, W.B. and Lubbock, G. (1979). 'How video tape has improved case conference'. *Geriatric Medicine*, 9, 3

4 THE DAY HOSPITAL

J.S. Tucker

Perhaps the first question to ask when considering establishing a
geriatric day care service is: 'What would a day hospital do for my area?'
The answer will depend to some extent on the nature of the community
which the day hospital is to serve. In a rural area where the provision of
day care by social services is minimal, the emphasis may have to be on a
'custodial' service. In a large town where the local authority runs day
centres which are able to cater for the essentially 'social' need, and where
there are day care facilities for psychogeriatric patients, and for the
younger disabled, it may well be possible to concentrate on a rehabilitation
orientated service with a high turnover.

In practice, the geriatric day hospital is likely to fulfil both custodial
and remedial roles. Reading through the literature covering 30 years of
experience with the concept of a hospital without beds for the elderly,
it is possible to trace the development of a more 'therapy'-orientated
approach. Many of the early descriptions emphasised maintenance of
patients in the community and advocated caution in discharging them
from day care. The more recent literature tends to favour concentrating
on remedial therapy, with suggestions that duration of attendance
should be carefully restricted. However, most units seem to find a
compromise between the two extremes. A small core of long-term
attenders may be accepted while the majority of patients attend only
for a limited period, for a clearly defined course of treatment. That this
blend is possible is well exemplified by the St Thomas's geriatric day
hospital, London. The unit was developed jointly by the local authority
and the health authority, and accepts day care clients from the social
services department of the former, and day hospital patients from the
geriatric unit of the latter. Such jointly-funded ventures are few in
number, but the advent of joint planning may allow for others in the
future.

Pathy (1969) has described the development of three complementary
geriatric day hospitals in Cardiff. One is associated with the acute
assessment unit and offers a diagnostic service with a great deal of
medical input and ready access to investigation facilities; the second is
part of a hospital where the emphasis is on rehabilitation, and hence
offers mainly remedial therapy; and the third, associated with a long-stay

58

hospital, offers custodial or social day care to patients who are too disabled for local authority units on a long-term basis. In a major city, the development of more than one day hospital, with differing approaches, may be better than concentrating all day care at one site, when the unit may become too large to be viable.

The Size of the Unit

These general points lead us on to a consideration of the design of the day unit. It is unlikely that any team planning a day hospital will be given *carte blanche* in this respect, but the importance of careful attention to design cannot be over-emphasised. The size of the unit may be dictated by availability of space, but most geriatricians seem to agree that 30 places is about the maximum. More than this and the day hospital becomes impersonal, the staff being unable to get to know their patients. It has been argued (Martin and Millard, 1976) that the smaller the day hospital, the more likely it is to function as a rehabilitation unit. These authors studied three day hospitals – the smallest, with twelve places, had a mean duration of attendance per patient of 5.5 weeks, and over two-thirds of patients achieved the objective of referral; the largest, with 28 places, had a mean duration of attendance of 15.1 weeks, and less than one-fifth of the patients achieved the aim of referral. On the other hand, a day hospital can be too small to be economically viable – in our analysis of the costs of day hospital care (Brocklehurst and Tucker, 1980), the small day hospital was significantly more expensive than the large unit. Around 30 places seems to me to be optimal.

Design

Virtually any accommodation can serve as a day hospital provided there is one good-sized room, and toilet and bathroom accommodation. Many successful day hospitals use adapted accommodation and I have heard at least one geriatrician express a preference for a good old hospital hall to house his day unit. However, fewer staff working in adapted premises express satisfaction with their work than in purpose-built accommodation, and certainly there are few old hospital buildings which can be adapted to provide nursing and remedial therapy areas to everyone's satisfaction.

Many different designs are available for a purpose-built day hospital, but the basic requirements are the same. A day hospital should have its own entrance, with good access for ambulances, and preferably a canopy to protect patients from the weather. There should be a reception area with cloakroom and storage area for walking aids, etc., and a good-sized sitting area. A separate quiet room is much appreciated, and a separate dining room with its own servery is preferable to having the sitting area double as a dining room. There should be adequate areas for physiotherapy and occupational therapy, with the emphasis on exercise areas in the former, and activities of daily living (ADL) assessment facilities in the latter.

Treatment and consulting rooms should be separate from the main areas, and adequate in number, the 'occasional' visitors to the day hospital such as the chiropodist and optician not being forgotten. The provision of an enema room apart from the general nursing treatment is favoured by most nursing staff.

There should be a good-sized room for meetings, conferences and teaching, and a room set aside for interviewing. Finally, the requirements of the staff for cloakroom and changing facilities, and a rest room, should not be forgotten.

The two most frequent complaints heard in purpose-built day hospitals are lack of storage space, with consequent clutter limiting the use of treatment areas, and inadequate attention to detail — incorrect height of windows, toilets unable to accommodate wheelchairs, and so on. Careful planning, by the whole team, is necessary.

The first purpose-built day hospital, at Cowley Road, Oxford, and several early day hospitals were built on the 'race-track' principle of having an endless corridor surrounding treatment areas where confused patients could wander without fear of getting lost. There is now less emphasis on the need to provide facilities for ambulant confused patients in a geriatric day hospital, but many subsequent designs have been modifications of this basic idea. A more recent tendency has been to have large open-plan areas used for sitting, dining, physiotherapy and occupational therapy, but these can be of a size that is rather daunting to patients, unless skilfully divided.

Some purpose-built units form the ground floor of a modern ward block and their design is dictated by the design of the wards — usually an open-plan area where the bed bays would be, and treatment rooms and offices down the other side.

Whatever the design, however, the most successful units seem to be those where the architect and the geriatric team have got together on the plan from the outset, and paid due attention to detail.

Transport

At a very early stage in the planning of a day hospital service, consideration must be given to the provision of transport. In the past too many day hospitals have been built and then run half-empty, because adequate ambulances and crew were simply not available to service them. With improved liaison this should not happen, but it is undoubtedly true that the success or failure of a day care service depends to a great extent on the adequacy of its transport.

Ideally a day hospital should have its own transport service with a permanent staff of drivers. There should probably be a variety of vehicles available to provide for patients with variable degrees of disability — from the chairfast patient who should be transported in his own chair, to the ambulant patient who can easily manage a journey in an ambulance car. In practice, the only vehicles available are often multi-purpose vehicles which are designed with the emphasis on accident and emergency work. 'Sitting'-type vehicles, with space for a wheelchair, and a tail lift, are best for the majority of patients. The larger buses are unsuitable, however, since the travelling time for more than 8-10 pick-ups can become unacceptable. Ambulance drivers have different views on the ideal day hospital vehicle, but most would agree that some variety and flexibility is desirable.

The idea of a team of ambulance personnel who work permanently on day hospital runs has its attractions, but is probably not practicable in most areas. It is perhaps more important that drivers on day hospital runs should not be concurrently standing-by for accident and emergency work. Where this is so, the number of patients who, at the last minute, cannot be transported to day hospital tends to be unacceptably high.

The use of part-timers, or even volunteers, to transport reasonably ambulant patients has been successfully explored in some day hospitals, but discussion on the role of such ancillary workers with the ambulance service will be necessary, and reliable people may not be easy to recruit. I know at least one day hospital where all patients are transported by retired part-timers using their own cars, but this obviously restricts the type of patient who can be brought in.

The majority of staff working in geriatric day hospitals cite transport as their biggest single problem. Complaints of late arrivals, early departures, and unacceptably long journey times are, unhappily, very frequent. Surprisingly, however, most patients seem to enjoy their ride to the day hospital (Brocklehurst and Tucker, 1980). Perhaps this lends some support to the suggestion (Arie, 1975) that 'transport-therapy' —

jogging the patient along in the ambulance for several hours, with a break at a café, might have a part to play in day care! Certainly, the journey is an important part of the day, and ambulance drivers are an important part of the team. The link which they are able to provide between home and hospital should be appreciated and utilised, and representatives of the ambulance service should be involved in discussions with the staff of the day hospital.

Staffing the Day Hospital

The staffing of day hospitals has been the subject of some debate. Martin and Millard (1978) have suggested that results—in terms of turnover and hence, presumably, satisfactorily rehabilitated patients—improve as the proportion of remedial staff to nursing staff increases. Where nursing staff predominate, the day hospital is more likely to have an essentially custodial function. Recommendations have been made by the Wessex Regional Hospital Board (1972) for staffing a day hospital. One nurse for six day hospital places was suggested, but this is certainly more generous than the funded establishment in most units. The recommendation for remedial staff was two physiotherapists, two occupational therapists, and four aides for 30 places; and for social workers, one per 50 places. The same recommendations for remedial therapists were made by the British Medical Association (1976), but the BMA Working Party commented that these levels were unlikely to be achieved for some time. Not only are they greater than funded establishments in most departments, but recruitment is difficult and many units have vacancies for physiotherapists and, even more, occupational therapists. The shortage of remedial staff is such that there must surely be a strong case for greater involvement of nursing staff in rehabilitation. Despite the traditional emphasis on 'care', most members of the nursing profession are happy to encourage patients to do things for themselves, and following advice from remedial therapists can surely contribute a great deal. This brings us to the important question of 'territorial rights', and staff relationships. On the whole, I have been impressed by how well remedial and nursing staff work together, but occasionally disputes over who should take patients to the toilet, and the like, can flare up into real problems. It is important that all staff should have a clearly defined role in the day hospital, but equally important that there should be some flexibility. The key to harmonious teamwork is liaison between the different professional groups in the day hospital, and regular meetings for discussion are essential. These may simply be an extension of the case conferences, or a 'programming' session, but they are a *sine qua non* of a good geriatric service.

The amount of medical input required will depend on the policy of the day hospital. Most units rely for day-to-day cover on general practitioner clinical assistant sessions, and an active average size day hospital will need at least five such sessions. Junior hospital doctors may also be involved in clerking new patients, ordering investigations, and so on. The consultant's involvement also varies from one unit to another. Some consultant geriatricians have no direct clinical involvement in the day hospital whatsoever, but most would feel that they should review patients there, in addition to their administrative involvement. One consultant session weekly will usually be adequate.

I have little doubt but that those day hospitals where a whole-time clerical officer/receptionist is part of the team function at an advantage. All too often the ordering of ambulances and routine clerical work are carried out by the senior nurse in the day hospital, and this must be to the detriment of her primary role. A good clerical officer can contribute much to the smooth running of the day hospital and should be requested as part of the establishment from the outset.

Regular sessions from a hospital social worker who has particular responsibility for the day hospital are also highly desirable. Much of the work may be liaison with community-based colleagues, but unless the other members of the team have a particular social worker (who should, of course, be involved in case conferences) to whom they can relate and refer problems, then these problems are less likely to be tackled.

Other staff should have a regular commitment to the day hospital. The 'on-demand' chiropodist, speech therapist, dietician and so on are far less effective than those who work a regular session in the unit. A visit, even if it is only monthly, from an optician, and a dental surgeon, which can be relied upon, is worth far more than unspecified sporadic contributions. Many staff play an important part in the day hospital and the provision of facilities for a hairdresser, an art therapist, or a beautician might be considered. The intangible, but all-important, concept of teamwork, which involves respect for and recognition of the contribution of each member, is the strength of a good unit.

Who Should Be In Charge?

Who should actually be in charge of the day hospital? In a health district, it is most usual for one consultant geriatrician to undertake overall administrative responsibility for the day hospital, although most consultants prefer to retain clinical control of their own day patients. The question of who should be in charge of the day-to-day running of the day unit, however, is even more important. At most day hospitals, a nursing sister is seen as being 'in charge', although she has no real control over the running of the physiotherapy and occupational therapy departments. In a few units, a remedial therapist assumes the role of director, and this often works quite well. The best person to be in charge may well be the most suitable candidate available within the day hospital staff, regardless of the professional group to which he or she belongs. Sometimes a doctor who spends a good deal of time in the day hospital – usually a medical assistant, sometimes a clinical assistant or junior hospital doctor – is seen as being in charge; and where this is so, other staff may comment that they consider this to be the best arrangement. However, the arrangement which, in my experience, meets with most enthusiasm from all day hospital staff is where no one is seen as being in charge! Each senior professional worker looks after his own 'patch', and the smooth running of the department depends on a thoroughly reliable receptionist/clerk. The best solution for one unit may not be suitable for another, and a consensus decision for each unit is needed at the outset.

Relationship with other Divisions of the Geriatric Department

The relationship of the day hospital with other divisions of the geriatric service demands some consideration. It seems logical for a good purpose-built unit with adequate remedial therapy facilities to serve not only as a day hospital, but also as the rehabilitation centre for geriatric inpatients. The latter, if space is available, could even spend a substantial part of the day there, particularly when they are approaching discharge. They would be able to meet equally disabled day patients from the community, and hopefully be encouraged by them. Lack of space and facilities might prevent full integration of the day care service and the inpatient rehabilitation service; but a day hospital working in isolation from the wards is unlikely to realise its full potential as an active contributor to the geriatric service.

A few day hospitals also house outpatient clinic suites. It may be argued that a day at the day hospital, where convivial surroundings, lunch and tea are available, is preferable to attendance at a busy outpatient clinic. This can obviously only be considered where the day hospital is on a DGH (District General Hospital) site with access to radiology and other diagnostic facilities. Certainly the staff in the day hospital are more likely to be geared to the needs of the elderly than those working in a general outpatient clinic; and it may be easier to get an opinion from the physiotherapist or occupational therapist at the first consultation. However, day hospitals involved in day care, inpatient rehabilitation and outpatient consultations can become rather hectic, and an outpatient suite separate from, but adjacent to the day hospital, with access to the facilities of the latter when required, might be the best compromise.

Referrals

Referrals to the day hospital are usually from the consultant geriatricians, and may be from outpatients, domiciliary consultations or assessment visits, or patients about to be discharged from the wards. A few units have experimented with allowing general practitioners direct access to the day hospital, but where this has happened there tended to be complaints from the staff that many patients were referred inappropriately. This situation is perhaps to be anticipated from the results of a survey of general practitioners' views on the day hospital by Hildick-Smith (1978). She found a great deal of confusion amongst general practitioners about the distinction between a day hospital and a social day centre. Obviously a unit with facilities and staff for professional nursing, physiotherapy and occupational therapy should not be used purely as a day centre, and most geriatricians feel that they must screen referrals themselves. The same problem is likely to arise when paramedical community workers are invited to refer patients directly to a day hospital.

It is not, however, easy to define the 'right' sort of patient for the day hospital. McComb and Powell-David (1961) described four categories of day hospital patients:

> those who were alone by day and needed care; those who were lonely and had some physical or personality defect; those requiring prolonged rehabilitation; those who were pleasantly confused.

Pathy (1969) described the type of patients attending his day hospital, his approach being rather different:

> those needing hospital services, but not acutely ill, who had predom-
> inantly physical disabilities; those requiring detailed investigation;
> those discharged from hospital who required technical services and
> medical and nursing supervision for a while; inpatients ready to go
> home but worried about leaving hospital

Brocklehurst (1970) surveyed the opinions of geriatricians on the purpose of the day hospital and found that while they saw rehabilitation as being the most important function, physical maintenance was seen as being almost equally important. In our recent survey (Brocklehurst and Tucker, 1980), day hospital staff were asked to define the reason for attendance in randomly selected patients. Rehabilitation came out top of the list, but there was a significant number of patients attending for rehabilitation for periods far in excess of what would be generally regarded as fruitful. While staff had mixed views on maintenance therapy, it seemed to us that this was in practice a very important function in most day hospitals. Further, there was a number of patients for whom no clearly defined reason for attendance was forthcoming.

It is important not only to formulate general guidelines for the sort of referrals which will be accepted by a day hospital, but to define clearly the purpose of attendance of each patient. Only then can rational decisions on progress be made, and best use be made of what is almost certain to be a scarce facility.

A clearly defined reason for attendance is also necessary if treatment is to be properly planned. Generally the referring doctor will outline the kind of treatment he has in mind in his initial referral — and some day hospitals have instigated referral forms for this purpose. If a patient is to get an individually planned treatment programme, then some kind of programming meeting of the team, on a regular basis, may be the most efficient way of doing this. A few day hospitals seem to offer all patients a uniform package of treatment, regardless of diagnosis or prognosis, and this is surely to be decried.

The need for regular review of patients is also obvious. Most con-
sultants hold case conferences at which the aims of treatment and the extent to which these are being realised are discussed by the team, but there is a tendency for patients not to be present at these sessions. Staff cannot adequately represent the patient's viewpoint, and my own practice is to see each patient under discussion after each member of

the team has described his or her progress, as part of the case conference.

Despite the demand, however, very few day hospitals have a waiting list for attendance. Geriatricians generally feel that long waiting lists are an admission of defeat, and are keen to keep the turnover such that admission to day hospital treatment can be on demand.

The patients who are likely to need long-term day hospital support fall into three categories:

> those who are alone by day and have significant physical disability such that care is needed; those alone by day who are significantly demented; those in either of the above categories who are not alone, but whose relatives or carers need a break from the burden of providing care.

Only where the disability is severe should patients in these groups be accepted for long-term day hospital care. The milder degrees of physical and mental infirmity can be adequately coped with in local authority day care, provided this is available.

Most geriatricians are agreed, also, that patients suffering predominantly from dementia should not attend the geriatric day hospital. The needs of the ambulant confused patient are quite different to those of the physically disabled, and it is generally felt that the two groups should be cared for in separate establishments. If there is no psychogeriatric day care facility, then a policy decision will have to be made at the outset whether ambulant demented patients will be accepted at the day hospital or not. Adequate links with the psychogeriatric service and with the local authority day care service are therefore very important. In general, day hospital staff, especially on the nursing and social work side, have quite good links with community services, but there is a need in many areas for a clearly defined policy of admission which is accepted by both the geriatric unit and the social services department for the various day care establishments available.

The Patient's Day

The structure of the patient's day varies from one day hospital to another. The most common pattern is for a morning drink to be available on arrival, followed by therapy—nursing treatment, remedial therapy, or medical review—on an individual basis. Lunch may be at one or two sittings, and therapy may continue in the afternoon.

Afternoons are the most popular time for group therapy, and a post-prandial rest seems to be common, and appreciated by patients. A frequent complaint made against day hospitals is that patients have too little to do, and spend too much of their time just sitting around, staring into space. Our survey of patients' views (Brocklehurst and Tucker, 1980) suggested that this is an unusual finding—most patients were satisfied with the structure of their day, and the free time allowed for quietly resting in a chair, doing nothing in particular, was generally appreciated. The correct balance will vary from one patient to another, and the need to provide an individual programme for each patient is apparent.

Most of the patients interviewed in our survey saw the purpose of the day hospital as did the staff, and cited therapy as the reason for their attendance. In the main, they enjoyed attending the day hospital and this was generally for the social outlet which it gave to them. There is no doubt that many patients fear discharge from day hospital, and a system whereby they can be transferred to social day care smoothly when their treatment is over is highly desirable.

On the other hand, patients' relatives saw the day hospital much more as a social facility than a therapeutic one. There was a good deal of confusion amongst them about the function of the unit, and I have no doubt that there is scope for much better liaison between the hospital, and the relatives or 'carers'. At least one day hospital holds regular evening meetings for relatives, and several units have designed handouts explaining the function of the unit. Patients' relatives are really members of the caring team, and efforts to gain their active co-operation can only be beneficial.

Liaison with the General Practitioner

So far little mention has been made of general practitioners; yet day hospital patients remain under the care of their family doctors throughout the period of their attendance. Perhaps the most important question is who should be responsible for prescribing when a patient is attending a day hospital. Some units stick rigidly to the principle that only a general practitioner should prescribe, and write to him advising any changes which medical staff at the day hospital have suggested. Others 'take over' the function of prescribing, but most steer a middle course, and prescribe short-term supplies of new medications, with a letter to the general practitioner informing him of the suggested change. Whatever system is decided upon, the need for adequate liaison is obvious. Some day hospitals have experimented with the use of drug cards, which should be kept up to date by both day hospital medical staff and general practitioners. These 'co-operation cards', as they are known in one day hospital, can be very useful, but can, of course, fail if patients forget them, or doctors do not keep them up to date. Ideally, general practitioners should be involved in other decisions made about their patients at the day hospital, and at least one unit has attempted to encourage this by holding the weekly case conference over lunchtime, and inviting doctors whose patients are to be discussed to come along. A buffet lunch is provided, and the support from local doctors is extremely good. There is certainly a good deal of interest in day care amongst general practitioners—many admit to knowing little about their local day hospital, but are keen to learn more (Hildick-Smith, 1978).

A Teaching Role

Finally, the use of the day hospital as a potential teaching facility deserves mention. In teaching hospitals, attendance at case conferences by medical students is a useful way of demonstrating the function of the geriatric team; and students of physiotherapy and occupational therapy can gain useful experience in the day hospital. The potential for training student nurses where there is a school of nursing is at present under-exploited. There must surely be a strong case for a short period spent in the day hospital as part of a secondment to geriatric nursing.

There are many different ideas about how a day hospital should be designed, and what it should do. Probably no two units are identical in their approach. However, there is general agreement on their value as part of the service—Brocklehurst (1970) found that only 4 per cent of geriatricians felt that day hospitals were of little or no value. Careful planning, bearing in mind the needs of the area, can result in a day hospital which effectively complements inpatient and community services, and is much appreciated by patients.

References

Arie, T. (1975). 'Day care in geriatric psychiatry'. *Gerontologia Clinica*, 17, 1, 31
British Medical Association, Board of Science and Education (1976). *Report of the Working Party on services for the elderly*. BMA, London

Brocklehurst, J.C. (1970). *The Geriatric Day Hospital. London.* King Edward's Hospital Fund for London

Brocklehurst, J.C. and Tucker, J.S. (1980). *Progress in Geriatric Day Care.* King Edward's Hospital Fund, London

Hildick-Smith, M. (1978). Paper presented at the Autumn meeting of the British Geriatrics Society, October, London

Martin, A. and Millard, P.H. (1976). 'Effect of size on the function of three day hospitals; the case for the small unit'. *Journal of the American Geriatrics Society*, 24, 11, 506

McComb, S.G. and Powell-David, J.D. (1961). 'A Geriatric day hospital'. *Gerontologia Clinica*, vol. 3, 3, 146

Pathy, M.S. (1969). 'Day hospitals for geriatric patients'. *Lancet*, ii, 533

5 THE HOSPITAL UNIT

R. Bailey

An early motto of the pioneers of geriatric medicine was that 'The best is not good enough for our patients'. Today the opportunity to establish a service with totally new resources falls to few, but all have the chance to develop some parts of their service. The developments undertaken will depend largely upon the facilities inherited, the availability of finance and the support of local management committees. This chapter concentrates on the development of the ward facilities within the geriatric service.

Design of a Hospital Unit

It is assumed that the unit is to be provided on the site of a hospital which already has all the necessary auxiliary services required for running a hospital, e.g. administration, laundry, canteen, accommodation for nurses, kitchen for the supply of patients' food, etc., and that the unit will have access to them as well as to the main remedial departments of occupational therapy, physiotherapy and speech therapy. Outpatient facilities must be available both for new patients and for the follow up of patients discharged from the wards. Facilities for specialist services such as chiropody, dentistry, dietetics, audiometry and ophthalmology should be available to patients within the unit and to those attending outpatients. If they do not already exist they can be conveniently sited within the day hospital (Chapter 4).

Access to the Unit

Elderly people have elderly relatives and it is, therefore, necessary that consideration should be given to ease of access to the department. Many visitors have to arrive by public transport, some arrive by private car or on foot. A covered drive and in-and-out vehicle waiting area should be provided with a canopy over the entrance, to give protection against the weather. Outpatients and patients attending the day hospital will arrive mainly in ambulances and these will probably have to use the same alighting and waiting facilities as those bringing patients for admission.

There should be a reception and information desk in the entrance hall of the unit to deal with all patients and visitors. Clear signposting must be provided to all wards and departments and the signposting should be in sufficiently large letters for people with poor vision to read. Waiting facilities must be provided near the entrance for those awaiting transport or for visitors.

Ward Design – General

The design of the ward will be dependent upon whether the ward already exists or whether it is purpose built. In England the tradition is of 'Nightingale' wards which essentially provide a dormitory area of beds running up and down opposite sides of a long ward, with lavatory and bathing facilities at one end. It is argued that the advantage of a ward of this type is that the patients can be easily observed at a glance, that they are not isolated and that they can draw a nurse's attention easily; patients are also reassured by having other patients close at hand. It is also argued that there is more privacy for conversation between patients and relatives in a large ward than in a 4- 6-bedded bay (one is more easily overheard in a small room than amidst the general hubbub of a large ward). These advantages, however, are outweighed by the disadvantages: one noisy patient disturbs all the others; it is not possible to barrier nurse and there is no privacy for those who really want to be isolated. In addition mixed-sex nursing, which may have a morale boosting affect, is impossible even with the very highest nursing standards. Toilet facilities are often inadequate. The lavatories are usually at the end of the ward and the disabled patient, whose mobility is poor and bladder control unstable, may spend a disproportionate amount of time going to and fro, or, worse, may give up the struggle with resultant distress to himself and the nursing staff.

An ideally sized ward would accommodate 20-22 patients. If any larger, it is difficult for staff to get to know the patients. Consideration should be given to the grouping of patients; for example, the use of one ward solely for stroke rehabilitation. This ward would need extra space for physiotherapy and occupational therapy. One ward might be set aside for the joint assessment of the elderly confused patient, with the bed allocation shared between the consultant in psychiatry and the consultant in geriatric medicine. Wards are preferably divided up into 4-bedded and 6-bedded bays with some single rooms and some double rooms; in this way males and females can be segregated in sleeping areas but still meet in day areas. Some single rooms allow flexibility of use. Double rooms also enable married couples to be accommodated. All wards which have facilities for both male and female patients should have ancillary toilet facilities designed accordingly.

Comments on Ward Design

Bed Areas

Where a Nightingale ward is being adapted for use, 4- or 6-bedded bays can be formed by dividing the ward with low-level partitions, solid up to about 3-4 ft from the floor with glass above this and provided with curtains. This allows greater observation when the curtains are open and privacy when the curtains are drawn. The majority of single rooms should be sited so that they can be seen from the nurses' station, but in order to keep the wards as compact as possible, a certain number could be sited at the far end of the ward for the more independent patient who is getting to the stage where he is about to be discharged home. Ideally all single rooms should have an *en suite* lavatory and washing facilities. The rooms should have large observation panels, which can be closed off by curtains when nursing procedures or medical examinations are being carried out. In the multi-bedded areas curtains should surround each bed to give the same privacy but should not be suspended from the ceiling which would cut out all natural daylight when they are drawn. There should be sufficient space around each bed for a patient to be able to sit in a chair and to be manoeuvred in and out of a wheelchair where necessary. The DHSS recommends that there should be 60 sq ft of floor area per bed. Easy access to toilets must be provided from all bed areas; space for sitting and dining should either be contiguous to the bed areas or provided in separate rooms. All patients should have individual mobile combined lockers and wardrobes.

Some physiotherapy and occupational therapy space, containing wall bars and parallel bars sited opposite a full-length mirror, should be provided around the bed areas, perhaps in the corner of the ward or in a day room, if access to the therapy department is difficult.

Day Spaces

A day room should be provided for each ward and should be sited so that the patients only have to walk a short distance to reach it. These rooms are suitable for watching television and for activities which might disturb other patients if they were carried out in the bed areas. It is preferable to have more than one day room to a ward, so that those patients who wish to have quietness whilst being up, or to watch television programmes, or to speak to their visitors, should be able to do so. It is important to remember that some of the patients will be extremely ill and noisy activities should be kept separate from them.

Ward Lighting

The day room should have low-level windows so that patients who are seated are able to look out. The windows should have adequate blinds to protect patients from direct sunlight and to darken the ward at night. Ideally, the lighting of the ward should be by natural sunlight and decoration should be chosen to make the ward as light and as cheerful as possible. Consideration should be given to the use of different coloured paint. At night, it is worth considering having light shining on the floor below bed level, rather than having a dim ceiling light lighting the whole ward. This enables patients who are getting out of bed to have sufficient light to see where they are going, without light shining in their eyes when trying to sleep.

Ward Decor

Attempts should be made to make the ward as home-like as possible; pictures should be provided on the walls to break the stark institutional decor and consideration should be given to using wallpaper in day rooms and to painting the ward in different colours. Facilities for cut flowers and pot plants are also needed. A long-stay ward is 'home' for those patients whose rehabilitation has been unsuccessful. These patients should be encouraged to have around them small personal possessions such as family photographs which help to maintain their identity in an otherwise impersonal environment.

Special Amenities

The provision of a hairdressing service to both inpatients and patients attending the day hospital boosts the morale of women of whatever age, and facilities for shaving and hairdressing for men should also be available. Consideration should also be given to the provision of other amenities, e.g. a daily newspaper service; a mobile library with large-print books; talking books for the blind; a mobile shop providing toiletries, fruit, chocolates and biscuits.

Sanitary Facilities

In designing these facilities, it is essential to remember the varying needs of patients. Various types and designs of lavatory and bathroom (containing bidet and wash-hand basins) should be provided. Some patients will need to be lifted from a wheelchair trolley into the bath, either manually or by a hoist. Standard bathrooms should also be provided to enable patients to take a bath independently. The standard bathrooms should have grab rails and other attachments. Facilities for some showers should also be provided. The patient should have space to sit whilst washing and the shower room should also be able to admit patients in a wheelchair. Shared areas should be curtained off for drying and dressing.

The control of incontinence in a ward is absolutely essential. In order to do this close proximity to lavatory accommodation must be provided for all ward areas. Outward opening or sliding doors should be wide enough to allow wheelchair patients to enter. All lavatories should be large enough for a patient to be assisted by one person if necessary, or to use a sanichair (Chapter 6). A certain number of larger lavatories are required for wheelchair patients and assistants where required. The more lavatories there are, the easier it is to maintain a high control of continence. Lavatory paper should be provided both on a roll and in sheets; this is important because a hemiplegic patient has difficulty in taking sheets of paper off a roll. Private washing cubicles for ambulant patients should be provided. The majority will wish to sit down and wash, and wash-hand basins and mirrors should be at a suitable height.

Nurses' Station

There should be one nurses' station per ward, situated centrally in such a position that the nursing staff can easily observe the whole ward.

Treatment Room

A treatment room should be provided near a clean utility room. Another large utility room should be provided for dirty sheets, clothing, etc.

Sister's Office/Doctors' Office/Interview Room

The ward should include several rooms which are private. One of these should be allocated as a sister's office and another for the doctors working on the ward so that they can interview relatives. Psychiatrists and social workers often complain bitterly that they have nowhere to go to interview patients on wards, when intimate details have to be discussed without being overheard by other patients.

A team approach to difficult problems of management has led to the development of case conferences which are often attended by a large number of staff. This requires a large room which may not be greatly used at other times and often the compromise of using the ward's day space is made. The use of the day room causes stress to the patients because the facilities which are for their use are taken up by staff.

Accommodation for Relatives

A room should be provided for overnight accommodation for relatives, when a patient is extremely ill. There should be toilet and washing facilities *en suite.* This room can be used for interviewing during the day.

Laundry

The problems of providing a personalised clothing service in hospital are innumerable (see Chapter 6). Every attempt must be made to make sure that the individual patient's clothes are labelled. Relatives should be encouraged to wash patient's clothing and return the clothes to the patient in hospital, where they can be stored in the patient's locker or wardrobe. Facilities must be provided for storing dirty articles of clothing. A washing machine and tumble dryer should be provided on each ward.

Ward Routine

It is traditional for acute hospitals to be run for the convenience of the staff, both medical and nursing, rather than for the comfort of the patients. Patients are woken early in the morning and given breakfast by the night staff who are about to leave. The day staff make the beds, wash the patients and prepare for the doctor's ward round, which is carried out in a silent ward with all the patients in bed. The patients spend their day lying in bed wearing night clothes and are available for dressing of wounds, investigations and teaching. Those who get up, sit in their clothes in the day room, but this makes it inconvenient for the consultant ward round. In the evening they are put to bed at an early hour by the day staff, ready for the arrival of the night staff. Meals are served at unusual times (breakfast at 8 a.m., lunch at 11.40 a.m., tea at 3 p.m. and evening meal at 6 p.m.). While this pattern may be appropriate for the acutely ill of any age including the elderly, patients with chronic disabilities, such as arthritis and stroke, require treatment directed at establishing independence in the activities of daily living and this should become an integral part of the ward routine.

Patients should be allowed to get up in their own time, dress at their own speed and be as independent as possible within the ward. This means that in addition to their traditional role, nurses have to assume the role of rehabilitation therapist in dealing with each individual patient. Hemiplegic patients must not be dressed by the nurse, but they should be supervised and encouraged to dress themselves. Arthritic patients should be encouraged to walk using a walking aid, and they should not be wheeled around in a wheelchair by the nurses. Patients with incontinence due to detrusor instability should be taken to the lavatory regularly instead of having bed pans or commodes brought to them. This approach may take longer than the alternatives but only in this way can the patient learn to regain his independence.

As this approach is more time-consuming, it is essential that the wards are fully staffed. A minimum staffing ratio of one nurse to every 1.25 patients is essential. With fewer nurses, short cuts are taken and rehabilitation suffers. Each patient has a different degree of disability and nursing staff need to bear this constantly in mind. Each requires a programme suited to his needs; patients need to know exactly what is expected of them and how they are likely to achieve independence. They should be told the expected length of their stay within the ward. It must also be explained to them that doing things for themselves is as much a part of their treatment as treatment with tablets. Patients, not particularly the elderly, often have fixed ideas about what goes on in hospital and expect to be nursed in the traditional model; they need careful handling to avoid resentment at the suggestion that they should help themselves.

Visitors

In general medical and surgical wards it is usual for visiting hours to be in the afternoon and early evening, limited to two adults at any one time and excluding young children. In geriatric medicine this inflexibility is inappropriate; visiting should be allowed at any time, so long as it does not conflict with the treatment of the patient and does not continue for so long that the patient is exhausted. In addition, young children are a source of pleasure to the elderly and, unless patients are suffering from an acute infectious illness, children should not be excluded from visiting.

The presence of close relatives in the rehabilitation department should be actively encouraged as they will be able to see the improvement the patient is making and learn how best to help the patient when he is discharged home.

Hospital Leaflet

It is worthwhile providing an explanatory leaflet which can be given to patients and relatives. The leaflet should contain details of ways of getting to the hospital by public transport, a map of the hospital showing the wards and a list of do's and don'ts. For example:

At the Beginning of Your Stay

1. A relation or close friend should accompany you when you are admitted to hospital, if at all possible, as the doctor and the nursing staff will want to meet them.
2. Please bring with you all the pills and potions that you have been taking prior to being admitted.
3. Clothes. Please bring (a) at least 2 sets of day clothes and underclothes (including ordinary walking shoes); (b) dressing gown and slippers and nightclothes. All these clothes should be labelled. Also bring flannel, soap, toothbrush, comb and brush, shampoo, box of tissues.
4. Please bring your walking frame, walking stick or wheelchair if you have one at home.
5. Valuables. You are advised that these should not be brought into hospital. There are facilities to keep a small quantity under lock and key.
6. Pension Books. These are usually only brought into hospital if there is no relation or friend to collect the pension. If the stay in hospital exceeds 8 weeks, the pension book must be returned to the Department of Health and Social Security.
7. If you live alone please bring the key to your own home.

During Your Stay

1. Telephoning. Enquiries about patients can be made at any time, but it would be helpful if one relative or friend could be responsible for keeping other members of the family informed of your progress, in order to reduce the number of enquiries.

2. Visiting. Routine visiting can take place at any time between (say) 10 a.m. and 8 p.m. At other times it is possible to visit with the ward sister's permission.
3. Relatives may be asked if they can help with the washing of patients' clothes. Dirty clothes are collected by the nursing staff and these can be taken away by relatives and friends.
4. In addition to meeting the doctor in charge of the ward at the time of admission, appointments to meet the doctor can be made via the sister or nurse in charge of the ward.
5. Social Services Department. Social workers are able to offer advice about living accommodation. They may visit you in hospital and make enquiries about this and about organising other services when you leave hospital.

Leaving the Ward

When you are about to leave hospital, notice will be given to friends and relations in good time. Any services which you had previously been receiving from the local authority can be restarted if necessary. When you leave hospital, you will be given a supply of the tablets that were prescribed for you by the doctor on the ward. If it is necessary for you to visit the hospital again as an outpatient an appointment card will be given to you and transport arranged if necessary. After you have been discharged home, the responsibility for your medical care returns to your general practitioner.

Ward Function

There are differences of opinion between departments of geriatric medicine as to whether and how patients should be 'streamed' (Chapter 3). In some, patients are admitted to any of the wards and remain there irrespective of their rate of progress. In others, the wards are divided into acute admission, rehabilitation and long-stay wards, with the medical, nursing and therapy staffing orientated to the different roles of the wards. This system is known as progressive patient care. Its antagonists argue that it has a damaging effect on the morale of those patients who are slow to improve and are transferred to wards in which there are increasingly more disabled patients. They also claim that it is better for the morale of the nurses when all the wards have an equal balance of disabled patients. The protagonists argue that whilst the acute assessment and rehabilitation wards may be run on the usual medical ward model with its emphasis on discharge, the long-stay wards have a different and specialised function (Chapter 3).

In a unit using a system of progressive patient care, admission to the long-stay ward will have followed a period of rehabilitation and assessment in the admission and rehabilitation wards. Several previous admissions to hospital may have occurred, and attempts to maintain the patient within the community, in his own home or Part III accommodation, will have been made. All the alternatives to long-stay care will have been fully explored and excluded. In practice the high quality of domiciliary services available within the UK has meant that only the most physically dependent and mentally frail require long-stay nursing care.

The emphasis of management must now be on caring rather than curing and the patients should be encouraged to make the ward their home and surround themselves with whatever belongings can be accommodated. The patients' day should be as informal as possible and they should be encouraged to partake in as many diversional activities as can be arranged. The help of voluntary groups can be enlisted to provide entertainment in the ward and for occasional outings to give a change of routine. Some units employ a Recreation Officer to co-ordinate the activities of voluntary helpers.

Occasionally there may be patients who improve after long periods in hospital. It is therefore impossible to be categorical that the long-stay ward will be their final home and that they will not regain sufficient independence to live in an old people's home or with a relative.

Ward Staff

The day-to-day management of inpatients is the responsibility of the junior doctors who are also involved in the day hospital and outpatient clinics. The consultant has overall responsibility for the patients and for making policy decisions. There are two ward sisters in charge of most geriatric wards in the United Kingdom and they are supervised by a nursing officer who is appointed to the whole department. The ward sister holds a key position as her attitude and philosophy can have a major effect on the morale of the junior nursing and paramedical staff. Detailed norms for medical, nursing and paramedical staffing are given in Appendix B of Chapter 2.

Adequate numbers of occupational therapists and physiotherapists are essential if a geriatric unit is going to achieve optimum results for its patients. Occupational therapy on the ward is usually limited to dressing practice and assessment of physical and mental disability. It is essential that occupational therapists and physiotherapists should work on the wards as well as in their respective departments. They must develop a close working relationship with nurses on the ward. Only in this way will the rehabilitation team reinforce each other's efforts in the area of activities of daily living. Most occupational therapists rightly feel that they should concentrate on rehabilitation and that diversional therapy should be done by voluntary workers or staff employed specifically for this purpose. The social worker is often the member of the team most familiar with a patient's home conditions and she will often have information of vital importance to the rehabilitation team.

Many hospitals have ward receptionists or hostesses, who may be paid or voluntary, to carry out administrative work which would otherwise be done by the nurses. They are general factotums, arranging appointments, fetching and carrying notes, and they may be used elsewhere in the hospital to usher or direct outpatients to their correct clinic. Whilst medical and nursing and therapy staff have the most prominent roles in the ward the patients often have close contact with the housekeeping staff who provide snacks and drinks, and with the porters who take patients to the therapy and X-ray departments. It is important that their attitude to the patients should be kind, tolerant and unpatronising.

6 WARD FURNITURE EQUIPMENT AND PATIENT CLOTHING

J. Andrews and L. Atkinson

In this chapter only items of equipment which are genuinely considered necessary to geriatric departments are discussed, but many of these items should of course be present in orthopaedic and general medical wards, where so many of the elderly and particularly the elderly handicapped are cared for. We are making suggestions on items of equipment on a 30-bed rather than a 24-bed ward complex. We think this is more realistic, although the latter is much more satisfactory from the nursing angle (DHSS, 1980).[1]

Structural Implications

Before discussing differing types of ward furniture, equipment and patient clothing, it is important to review some of the known problem areas associated with the structure of the ward. By so doing it may be possible to prevent commissioning teams making unnecessary mistakes when designing new or upgraded departments.

Flooring

There has been much debate over the use of polyvinyl chloride (PVC)/ linoleum or its equivalent versus carpeting, particularly in wards for the elderly. Some of the starkness of a ward is softened by carpet; noise, a constant factor in hospitals, is deadened when carpets are used. Although synthetic carpeting now available is not difficult to clean, advice to facilitate the cleaning of incontinence stains suggests that carpets should be of non-absorptive nylon, acrylic or polyester fabrics as they are the easiest to keep clean (Goldsmith, 1976). However, the difficulty of cleaning some carpets, the unsatisfactory manner in which carpet tiles ride up after minimum use, the obvious new patches seen where some of the carpeting has been replaced, due particularly to wear from beds and chairs, calls for a selective approach in their use.

Passages, single rooms and 2-, 4- and 6-bedded bays should have easy-care non-slip PVC flooring, whilst the day areas should be carpeted, thus facilitating the training of wheelchair and walking-aid users as well as attempting to give a more homely atmosphere. Floor surfaces show up dirt and mark less if a patterned surface is chosen. However, a chequerboard or herringbone pattern should be avoided as it can seriously disorientate the elderly with perceptual problems (Agate, 1969). An intermediate colour is best as light-coloured finishes mark easily with wheelchair tyres (Goldsmith, 1976).

Colour Schemes

Rigidly keeping to a single colour for the whole ward is bound to cause problems. It is better to produce a theme of several mutually blending colours to allow the furniture acquired later to blend with the colour scheme. Batches of dye for such items as curtains and chair covers are only on the market for a limited time before being replaced by those of a different hue. In order to help patient orientation in strange surroundings, toilet doors should be painted in the same bold colours throughout (Agate, 1969).

Storage

Nearly all geriatric departments, even those in new buildings, are found to have inadequate storage space. Adequate storage must be provided for wheelchairs at night, and space for hoists, sanichairs, commodes and walking frames must be planned during the design stage. A large storage area is needed for disposable bedpans in the sanitary annexe (DHSS, 1980), such bedpans being essential in geriatric departments. Enough space is necessary in the ward area for the remedial staff to keep a range of walking aids, early walking boots, below-knee irons, and eating and dressing aids. Sophisticated beds not currently in use also make great demands on storage space. In many newly designed wards individual lockers with hanging space are provided beside the washroom area, but this in no way obviates the necessity for a small locker with hanging space being placed next to each patient's bed for activities of daily living practice.

Design of Sanitary Annexes

In the planning stages, whether for a new unit or an upgraded unit, considerable thought must be given to their design (see Chapter 5, p. 75).

Television and Radio Connections

These should be available at each bed with ear pieces for sound. In addition, electrical socket outlets for shaving at the bedside should be available. Television and radio in the day rooms are for the benefit of the patients, not of the staff.

Piped Oxygen Inlets and Suction

Such facilities are needed for a proportion of the admission beds, and should not be denied to the geriatric unit.

Policies

A geriatric unit must not be allowed to stagnate — it must be encouraged to try out new equipment and therefore policies must be formulated in advance. This applies equally to a new ward or day hospital as to a renovated building. The commissioning team, and subsequently staff who will be participating in the use of the ward furniture/equipment and clothing, have to know where to seek information. Where practicable, specialised equipment should be bought after the unit has been running for a while, so that there can be staff involvement in purchase. If staff are not involved in the choice of equipment it will not be properly used (Andrews and Atkinson, 1978). So often ward furniture and equipment are used by different staff members at different times of the day, and failure to know who is responsible for reordering, replacing and repairing this equipment leads to a most unsatisfactory state of affairs.

When opened, new or upgraded wards or day hospitals usually gain much publicity. Everything is fresh, new and conforms usually in shape, size and colour. The same unit seen two years later can be a great disappointment: much equipment may be awaiting repair, the tasteful colour scheme may have been abandoned and there may be evident lack of pride in the staff who had initially tried their hardest to get modifications and/or repairs carried out. Repeated failure can result in an attitude of 'it's no good trying to do anything, nothing will be done'.

Financial Policy

Adequate funding must be available for initial capital spending and to provide equipment during the first two years after commissioning when staff have had time to discuss and try out equipment. Revenue monies must also be available annually for maintenance and replacement when needed of existing equipment in addition to purchasing proven satisfactory new equipment. By this means, spending sprees on unsuitable and/or unnecessarily expensive equipment at the end of each financial year can be prevented.

Maintenance Policy

This must be clearly stated in writing so that all staff are aware of the necessary procedures. One person should be responsible for the equipment on the ward and one method available for notifying faults and problems (Andrews and Atkinson, 1975). The person responsible for deciding which items of equipment should be repaired and which should be replaced should be known to all staff. Equally, someone should be responsible for recording the time taken between request for repair and its implementation and likewise be responsible for reporting equipment lost, stolen or mislaid. If equipment is clearly marked with the ward name or number, it is less likely to go astray. It can be of advantage to enter into a maintenance agreement for some items of sophisticated equipment already bought to be serviced by the manufacturer. This ensures that expertise which is not necessarily at hand in the individual hospital is available for their maintenance.

Policy on Assessment of New Equipment

Many enterprising manufacturers loan expensive items of equipment to units for trial periods to increase sales. A loan system should be encouraged, but staff must be aware that the same or similar pieces of equipment may be produced by more than one firm (Andrews and Atkinson, 1978). Therefore, a small team of medical, nursing and remedial staff should represent the unit, making sure that visits to aids centres (Disabled Living Foundation, 1980) and hospital equipment exhibitions are regularly undertaken and also that visits are arranged to units using new equipment (Andrews and Atkinson, 1976). Regular full geriatric unit meetings, specifically devoted to discuss equipment, should take place to keep all staff informed of new developments. These meetings should allow representation from nursing officers on night duty to ensure that subsequent teaching of night staff on the use of new sophisticated equipment can occur. It is also important to have reports from the night staff concerning items needing repair. Hiring is another way of assessing the suitability of equipment – many firms offer this service, and of course maintain the equipment whilst it is on hire.

Policy on Education of Staff

Not only do staff need practical teaching on new sophisticated equipment, but they also require written instructions. Staff frequently move from ward to ward and the beds/hoists/chairs can differ considerably on different wards. If the instruction sheets are available in a loose-leaf folder, relevant data of maintenance dates and the frequency with which worn parts need replacing can be recorded. With some items of equipment, it is useful to have the instructions incorporated on the equipment itself.

Items of Furniture/Equipment

Any innate desire for uniformity and symmetry in choosing equipment should be resisted. It is essential that there is a wide range of equipment to match the different shapes and sizes of patients who over the years may develop different deformities.

Beds and Their Accessories

It was perhaps unfortunate that the UK Working Party on specifications for a general-purpose bedstead (King's Fund Working Party—*Design of Hospital Bedsteads*, 1967) did not take account of the development of bed design in Continental Europe and North America. Since 1967, British bed manufacturers have been in practice limited by the King's Fund specifications and encouraged to believe this should be provided for all hospital bed users, and the British Standards Institution specifications of a fixed-height bed—still set at 60 cm (24 inches) to the mattress frame.

The use of contour beds (Figure 6.1) for patients' comfort and the prevention and treatment of pressure sores has been advocated since the 1960s (Gainsborough, 1967; Andrews, 1970; Andrews, 1971a), yet only recently have British firms been manufacturing and displaying such beds at equipment exhibitions. Most of the beds on display are still a 3-section rather than a 4-section design. Of course, there is an important place for the King's Fund general-purpose bedstead but its use should be limited in each ward to patients needing much nursing attention but not in danger of contracting pressure sores.

There is a wide choice of beds available to equip a unit. All units require a variety of beds, many of which can be simple height-adjustable beds whose lower cost can offset some of the essential but expensive beds required to prevent or treat pressure sores. Fortunately, some of the newly produced contour beds are available in this lower price range.

General Points. (a) Every bed should be *height adjustable* if the bed is to be used for transferring from bed to wheelchair, sanichair,

Figure 6.1: (Above) Shearing Strain Produced on Buttocks and Heels on a Conventional Bed. (Below) Diagram of 4-sectioned (Contour) Height-adjustable Bed

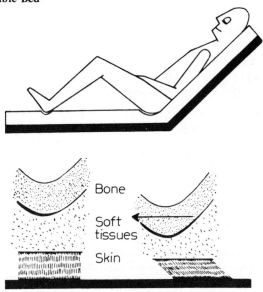

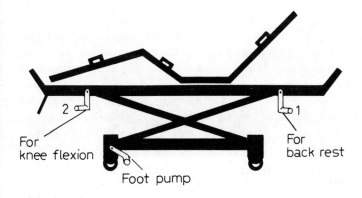

commode or walking aid.

(b) A safe and simple system of *braking* is required (Atkinson, 1971).

(c) All beds should be capable of having *safety sides* attached to them which can be easily stored, are three-quarter length and not too high

and which do not hurt nurses' hands on bedmaking (British Geriatrics Society and Royal College of Nursing, 1975).
(d) The beds should be designed to take *drip poles, overhead pullies* and a few should have facilities for *traction* for use in combined orthopaedic/geriatric wards.

Sophisticated Beds. A height-adjustable contour bed with the mattress base hinged in four sections is preferred to a mattress base in three sections; all beds of this type must be height adjustable. *Turning and tilting beds* (Figure 6.2) with a lateral tilt are also of significant help with pressure sores, these beds being designed originally for spinal injury patients. These beds can also be placed in the Trendelenburg and reverse Trendelenburg positions.

Figure 6.2: Turning and Tilting Bed with Safety Side in Position

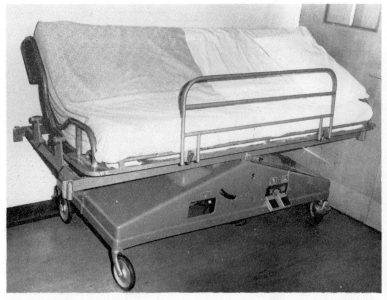

Supplier: Egerton & Co. (Hospital Equipment) Ltd, Tower Hill, Horsham, West Sussex RH8 7JT.

True flotation water beds (Figure 6.3) as opposed to those which are only water-filled mattress envelopes, are good for healing pressure sores. However, care must be taken in choosing the right patient for them as problems can arise for the physiotherapists and nurses when

Figure 6.3: Position of Patient within the Nylon-fabric Envelope of a Flotation Water Bed

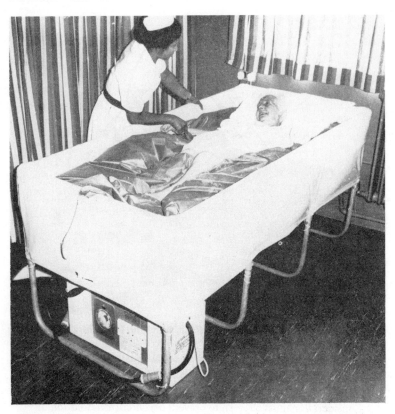

Supplier: Paraglide Ltd, Wren Nest Mill, High Street West, Glossop, Derbyshire SK13 8EZ.

trying to mobilise patients from this type of bed. A new model with castors is now available and makes transfer of the bed from ward to ward easier. The *Clinitron* air fluidised bed also provides flotation by blowing thermostatically controlled air through microspheres and is also effective in the prevention and treatment of pressure sores.

The highly effective *contour low air loss bed* (Figure 6.4) is often unfortunately, on account of cost, restricted to those patients who are very ill and therefore in danger of contracting sores or to those who have serious sores on admission (Andrews and Atkinson, 1978). These beds should be much more freely available. A new model is available

Figure 6.4: Low Air Loss Bed in Contour Position with Console (Safety Sides Attached)

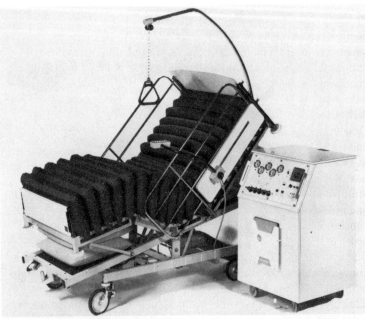

Supplier: Mediscus Ltd, 7 Westminster Road, Wareham, Dorset EH27 7SP.

which can be placed on an ordinary hospital bedstead.

The weight of sophisticated beds. Water, sand and microsphere-type beds may be too heavy for existing ceilings in old buildings.

Consideration must be given to prevent *psychological isolation* of patients. Some sophisticated beds, although aiding the healing of sores, prevent patients from sitting up and orientating themselves, thus adding to any feeling of isolation they may have. Therefore, when selecting from the wide variety of anti-pressure sore beds available those combined with a contour mechanism should be used when clinically suitable.

Recommendations. In any ward catering for the admission of very ill elderly patients it is essential to have a number of sophisticated patient support systems (Andrews and Atkinson, 1978). On admission wards at least a dozen beds should be suitable for the prevention and treatment of pressure sores, including perhaps at least one low air loss bed, one flotation water bed, one air fluidised bed and one tilting and turning bed, the remainder being height-adjustable contour beds. The other beds in the ward should be height-adjustable and should probably include four 'King's Fund' bedsteads.

Beds in Continuing-care Wards. Contour beds may add to patients' comfort, but pressure sores should not generally occur in long-stay patients with an intact sensory system, and therefore sophisticated anti-pressure sore beds should rarely be needed. All beds should of course be height-adjustable.

Mattresses and Covers. Research at the Biomechanical Research and Development Unit (Shaw, 1979) has been investigating mattress design and mattress covers. The usual hospital mattress (BSI recommendation at 14 cm deep) contained in a tight cover was thought by them to be one of the precipitating factors in the development of pressure sores. Multiple layers of sheets and/or tight tucking in of both under-layers and over-layers adds a further hazard and increases pressure. Their conclusions favour a Polyfloat mattress (the upper layer being cut in order to form a number of almost independent foam blocks, Figure 6.5) with a soft, loose-fitting mattress cover which can be used on conventional or contour beds. A change from a typical foam mattress with a tight-fitting cover to a Polyfloat mattress with its loose cover allowing for a covering sheet in both cases has been shown almost to halve heel pressures.

Other Anti-pressure Sore Devices. Many items other than beds have been designed to prevent sores. They include gel, cushions, ripple mattresses, and sheepskin rugs and bootees. The latter have been found of definite value in the prevention of heel sores. As ripple beds are often used incorrectly, their efficacy is difficult to judge objectively (Bliss, 1978).

Continental Quilts/Duvets. The freedom produced by a duvet is an asset in reducing the likelihood of flexion contractures at the ankle and makes it easier for the patients to follow their physiological instinct to turn frequently, thus helping to reduce the incidence of pressure sores. In emergencies, it is much easier to remove handicapped patients quickly by throwing aside a duvet rather than extracting them from under tightly tucked sheets and blankets. Duvets, commonly used in many countries, have now been introduced into many hospitals in the UK, having been approved by the appropriate Health and Safety Committees. As they have advantages from the aspects of patient

Figure 6.5: Polyfloat Mattress with Loose Mattress Cover

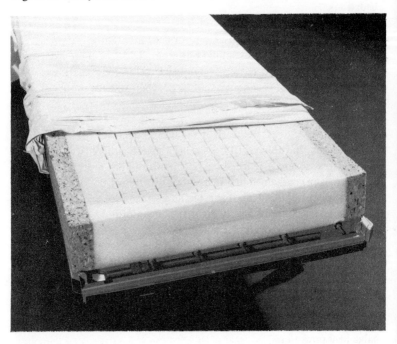

comfort, economics and fire risk, they should be much more widely used (Henderson, 1981).

Bed Cradles. Some patients will require bed cradles on admission, particularly stroke patients, those with peripheral vascular disease, leg ulcers and a proportion of patients suffering from rheumatoid arthritis. Cradles are often underused because they are cumbersome and difficult to store, but a folding cradle is on the market. Compactness is also an advantage because the use of bulky cradles can result in patients feeling cold. However, greater use of continental quilts should lessen the need for bed cradles in the future.

Cantilever, Height-adjustable Over-bed Tables. There is a wide range of over-bed tables available. The report of the Research Institute into Consumer Affairs No. 11 (1972) on over-bed tables made good recommend-ations. It must be decided before purchase whether the table is to be used solely over a bed or over a chair as well. If it is to be used over a chair, the base must not get in the way of the patient's feet or the chair legs. It must also be decided whether a drawer for personal belongings which incorporates a looking glass, is needed, and if so the model should allow room for knee clearance in bed.

Lockers

Bedside lockers should allow hanging space for personalised clothing and allow display of such items as personal photographs and cards. Continuing-care wards, not purpose-built with single rooms, can be divided with wardrobe-lockers acting as cubicle dividers (Andrews and Atkinson, 1978).

Adjustable Couches

To allow easier patient handling during examination, a height-adjustable couch is helpful both in the day hospital and in outpatients. The traditional high couch used with steps is unsuitable and potentially dangerous for many elderly patients with locomotor problems and poor sight (Andrews, 1969).

Chairs

When equipping each ward there must be a wide range of chairs available for use both beside the bed and in the day areas. A height-adjustable assessment chair is required which allows alteration of the angle of the seat and rake (Atkinson, 1971) to assist remedial staff to select the correct height and angle of the chair seat.

Chairs of different seat heights need to be available to match the individual requirements of the patients. Research on the ergonomic requirements of the population in general, and the elderly in particular, fortunately continues (Bramwell-Jones, 1968; Goldsmith, 1976). Mobile chairs will always be needed in all wards. They must have a safe braking system and easy to use foot-rests that fold away when not required.

General Points. (a) *Stability* is needed for patients such as hemiplegics with a one-sided thrust when attempting to stand up or sit down. (b) Well-positioned *hand grips* encourage patients to push themselves up with their hands when attempting to stand (Bramwell-Jones, 1968,) whilst (c) the *absence of a front cross bar* allows correct positioning of feet under the chair. (d) *Padded arm rests* lend comfort. Winged chairs should be bought and used sparingly. Although wings may be essential for some patients lacking head control, their overuse in an institutionalised setting diminishes visual and auditory contact.

The following suggestions may be useful for guidance. A chair chosen individually for each patient should be positioned by the bed, therefore 30 chairs of varying heights are needed. In the day room areas another 20 static chairs will be needed, again of varying design, with an additional 10 mobile chairs for transporting immobile patients from bed to day area to toilet. Specialised chairs which allow patients to be tipped back, thus preventing forward sliding, are an advantage for a few patients. However the angle adopted should always be the minimum tilt commensurate with safety (Andrews and Atkinson, 1978).

Transit Chairs

Each ward should have at least three transit chairs clearly marked with the name of the ward for movement to and from X-ray, occupational therapy and physiotherapy departments, thus preventing patients' personal chairs and the unit assessment chairs being taken from the ward and not returned.

Hoists

A booklet on preventing back strain in nurses emphasises the need for hoists (Royal College of Nursing, 1979). Recently the Disabled Living Foundation published a book on this topic which should be consulted by commissioning teams and readily available to all staff (Tarling, 1980).

It is important, once the hoists have been selected, that there should be regular and 'on-going' tuition of all staff on their safe use. Nursing and remedial staff should teach junior staff and students and should be encouraged to look for and report worn or cracked canvasses. It is essential to have a domestic hoist available for practice on the ward and for loan for trial periods at home.

Tables

Tables chosen for the dining area should be of differing heights and made to seat not more than four persons. Wheelchair users need a lower height (Goldsmith, 1976). In the remedial area some units find a height-adjustable table useful. The tables should also have well placed legs to allow ease of access, particularly for wheelchair users (Andrews and Atkinson, 1975/76).

Toileting

Ideally the patient should walk to the lavatory. If this is not possible a sanichair can be used by day and converted into a bedside commode at night. A disposable bedpan should be used as a last resort for the very ill or the very handicapped. The use of this type of equipment is closely linked with the overall policy of the unit to incontinence. Space must be allowed for storage of sanichairs and commodes. For those patients returning home who will need a commode at their bedside, there is a model on the market which has height-adjustable legs which can be attached to a bed.

It is important to purchase sanichairs which can be used as commodes when required and indeed even as a shower chair (Andrews and Atkinson, 1978). They help considerably where patients are rightly reluctant to open their bowels in a ward on a bedpan or commode because of the embarrassment of faecal smells and lack of privacy. Use of a sanichair encourages independence by re-establishing normal routine. Foot-rests that are fixed should be avoided – sliding or folding foot-rests prevent both patients and staff knocking their legs. The sanichairs must have a safe braking system to give confidence when the patient transfers and to prevent any movement once placed in position over the lavatory pan. Some sanichairs are self-propelling – another step nearer to independence for the patient (Figure 6.6).

Baths and Showers

Fortunately for nurses, height-adjustable baths, both UK produced and imported from Scandinavia and Holland, are now available (Figure 6.7a). When used in the low position they allow easier transfer for mobile patients and in the high position they prevent strain on nurses' backs while bathing patients. These new height-adjustable baths can be used with hoists for immobile patients. A recent advance for semi-ambulant patients is the Parker bath. This bath is height-adjustable and by opening the side allows easy patient transfer, negating the use of the hoist. Once the patient has entered the bath, this is reclined to produce immersion (Figure 6.7b). Each ward should have one bath that is height adjustable for bathing the heaviest immobile patient, as well as conventional baths and a walk-in sit-down bath for those with limited range of movement at the hips and knees (Andrews, 1971b).

Showers are not yet favoured by many elderly patients, but used with a shower chair they may in fact be very suitable for some. Showers should have controls accessible to the attendant, the shower head should not be fixed but have several different positions, and there should be a sloping floor to the drain, with no lip to impede a wheelchair.

Bathing Aids are supplied to patients in their own home by social services departments in the United Kingdom and should be present on

Figure 6.6: Self-propelling Sanichair/Commode Illustrating Individual Parts

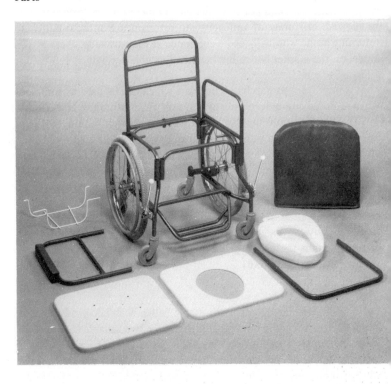

Supplier: F.J. Payne (Manufacturing) Ltd, Stanton Harcourt Road, Eynsham, Oxford OX8 1HY.

the ward to allow occupational therapists to try them out with patients and train both the patient and relatives in their safe use (Andrews and Atkinson, 1977). In addition to grab rails, over-bath boards, inner bath seats and non-slip mats or strips permanently put in the bath, should be available. For nearer simulation to a patient's own bathroom, the Activities of Daily Living (ADL) assessment bathroom in the occupational therapy department may well be used for training as well as assessing.

Basins should be of cantilever design to allow free access by wheelchair patients. There should be basins at different heights to help both ambulant and wheelchair disabled, with suitably-placed looking glasses.

Taps at the front of vanity units can help patients with limited reach, whilst lever taps will allow many with a poor grip greater

Figure 6.7a: Height-adjustable Bath Shown in High Position

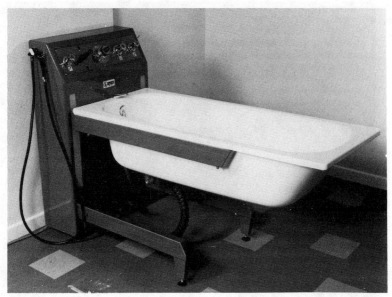

Supplier: Mecanaids Ltd, St Catherines's Street, Gloucester GL1 2BX.

independence (Goldsmith, 1976).

Equipment Used by Remedial Staff

Parallel Bars, Wall Bars and Practice Stairs. All three should be routinely available in the day hospital. In addition parallel walking bars and wall bars should be available in each ward which is carrying out physical rehabilitation. A Westminster plinth is a great asset and adequate numbers of walking sticks and frames of various heights must be available.

Eating Aids. Non-slip mats and special eating aids should be available where necessary.

Self-propelling Wheelchairs. Each unit needs a range of commonly prescribed wheelchairs for assessment and trial, and we recommend that one of each of these models supplied by the Department of Health be held:

8L Rear-propelling wheel ⎫	One model should have
8BL Rear-propelling wheel ⎬	capstan rings
8L Front-propelling wheel	

Figure 6.7b: Parker Bath

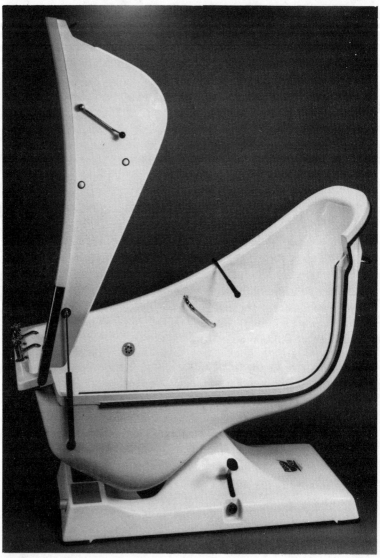

Marketed by: Parker Bath Developments, Sten Lane, Industrial Estate, New Milton, Hampshire BH2 5NN.

8L foot steering
One-arm propulsion chair
Recliner with elevating leg rests
Glideabout
Battery-operated chair

Personal instruction books (DHSS, 1979) and Ministry handbooks (DHSS, 1978) should be readily available to staff.

It is important that suitable wheelchairs are available for continuing-care patients to use in the garden. These chairs should be folding so that they can be placed in the boot of a car when the patient is being taken out by friends or relatives. These continuing-care patients are entitled to Department of Health wheelchairs if they are immobile. However, unless an individual patient goes out regularly, it is unnecessary for each to have his own wheelchair. Only those capable of propelling a chair need a self-propelling chair; for the remainder a 9L with soft cushion is generally suitable. Adequate storage space is again essential.

Miscellaneous

When considering ward furniture and equipment, it is all too easy to forget smaller items of equipment which give much comfort to patients and the absence of which can retard rehabilitation. Many pieces of standard equipment are often not available on geriatric wards, including such items as high/low reading ward wall thermometers, low reading clinical thermometers, and nail clippers.

Denture Holders. These should be kept as part of the ward stock and individually named for each patient. Checks should be made to ensure that denture cleansing solution and tooth brushes are available.

Spectacles and Hearing Aids. These should be labelled routinely on admission, and spare batteries for the latter should be available on the wards.

Linco Hearing Aids. These should be kept on each ward to help those with limited hearing. It greatly aids history-taking and allows those with hearing loss to participate in recreational activities.

Chair Weighing Machines. For accurate weighing of hemiplegic patients, under uniform conditions, a weighing machine incorporating a foot-rest is strongly recommended.

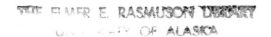

Foot-stools. Patients with oedematous legs, arthrodesed knees and other conditions causing incapacity will need to have their legs supported. For these patients, foot-stools which allow full support of thigh and calf and which adjust in height and angle to suit each individual chair height, are an asset. They allow the heel to remain free, thus preventing pressure. At least four are necessary in the ward.

Clocks and Calendars. Large clocks with suitable illumination placed in key positions in the ward complex encourage patient-orientation; likewise calendars can be of help.

Patient Clothing

The smooth running of a clothing policy is closely linked to the ward policy on incontinence. Unless a policy of habit training and use of protective clothing is in force, nurses will quickly deny incontinent patients underwear and discourage personalised clothing. Advice on an incontinence policy is given in the British Geriatrics Society and the Royal College of Nursing Booklet (1975).

Personalised clothing has been encouraged by the Department of Health and Social Security since 1972 (DHSS, 1972) and Hospital/ Health Advisory Service reports repeatedly recommend the implement-ation of personalised clothing schemes (Health Advisory Service Report, 1977). From every angle it is obviously much better for patients to have their own clothes chosen, maintained and supplied by themselves or their families (DHSS, 1977). The otherwise admirable report on the Bolton scheme (Hinchcliffe, 1980) appears to disregard this point, which had been advised in the Domestic Services Management Advice Notes (1977). Implementation of a personalised clothing scheme undoubtedly gives more work to the staff, but it encourages self-respect and individual-ity, and provides pleasure to the patients.

Many frustrations will be prevented if a clear clothing policy has been formulated. Responsibility for patients' clothing appears to be the most serious problem. If the clothing is lost or damaged, who is responsible? If relatives and friends feel the slightest doubt that patients' clothing could be mislaid, they will not co-operate and bring in further items. Under these circumstances a clothing policy is doomed to failure.

To be really effective a clothing policy must involve a variety of personnel.

Administrators can encourage the smooth running by supporting ward sisters or charge nurses when there is any loss of personal clothing. If this support is lacking, ward staff will be less than enthusiastic in encouraging patients to wear their own clothes. If is therefore helpful if the administrators can expedite the inevitable replacement of the few items of clothing lost. Their help is also needed in supplying finance for the ward pool of clothing and for keeping it 'topped up' when numbers dwindle due to wear and tear and/or loss.

Laundry Managers can help to implement the clothing policy. Either the laundry manager designates both equipment and staff in the main laundry to deal with personalised clothing, or laundry equipment is made available on the ward or in the unit as a whole, with staff designated to carry out this function (Hospital Advisory Service Report, 1969/70).

Supplies Officers have expertise in buying equipment and their specialist knowledge should be sought (King's Fund Centre Report, 1979).

Needleroom Staff must be closely associated with the geriatric department so that repairs to personalised clothing can be carried out quickly. In some hospitals they provide some means of identification of personalised clothing such as name tags (Hospital Advisory Service Report, 1976).

Nursing Officers hold a key position. They should encourage the use of personal clothing on their wards and should maintain close contact with the ward occupational therapist when specially designed clothing for patients with locomotor problems is required. Relations and/or friends will feel much more involved in the patients' treatment if written advice is given on suitable clothing and verbal explanations given if problems arise such as those occurring from delays in laundering.

Occupational Therapy Staff must give individual advice to patients, relatives and/or friends concerning the best use of the patients' own clothes in hospital. They should also give initial and 'ongoing' advice on suitable items for the ward clothing pool. Hospital clothing from such a pool will always be needed by a small group of patients – those newly admitted in an emergency awaiting their own clothing, those without family to maintain clothing, and those severely incontinent. For females, dresses in an easy button-through coat style, with fullness at the waist and long sleeves, in easy-care material and in several sizes, are recommended. Future generations may well prefer to wear slacks. Cotton underwear, hold-up stockings and open-back nighties are all required. Men need washable trousers, shirts, club coats/cardigans, underwear and open-back nightshirts in easy-care material and in different sizes. Socks should be kept to one colour for ease of pairing. With co-operation from the manufacturers, it is possible for those patients who initially need to make use of the pool clothing to use colours to form a colour code for sizing, e.g. green trousers, green check shirt and green night shirt indicates large size. It is not suggested that this scheme should be used for personal clothing for continuing-care patients whose own tastes must be catered for.

Ward Housekeepers. In the Bolton Area Health Authority this interesting post has been established (Hinchcliffe, 1980). Among other duties the ward housekeeper checks clean garments, stores them in patients' lockers and returns unserviceable garments for repair or disposal.

Footwear

Footwear is a separate problem. On admission to the geriatric unit many patients are found to be without shoes, having given them up because of such conditions as bunions, corns, metatarsalgia, oedema and uncut toenails. If surgical shoes are not needed, firm outdoor type shoes are required for retraining in walking and use with below-knee irons or calipers. Therefore, a policy concerning the provision of shoes is necessary and may involve using mail order firms or arranging for local shops to send in a representative. The social work department can sometimes provide finance for these items (Health Advisory Service Report, 1977).

Abuse and Non-use of Equipment and Clothing

This arises either because the right equipment is not known about, has never been ordered, has been broken and not repaired, or has been purchased in insufficient numbers. The staff may not have been trained in the appropriate use of the equipment concerned. Sometimes the items bought are unsuitable and have been ordered by staff with no knowledge of the subject. Under such circumstances, the equipment is rarely or never used to its full potential.

Chairs

The danger of excessive tilting and over-use of tilting chairs must be emphasised. Their misuse can give the patient a feeling of being 'captive', especially with the tray in position. Patients are unable to make use of appropriate proprioceptive stimulation from the soles of their feet, are visually placed in an unnatural position, and are more likely to suffer from postural hypotension on standing. Static chairs can be dragged from one place to another to move patients because of the lack of mobile chairs. Patients can be placed in chairs of the wrong height and the angle of the seat may be unsuitable. Trays attached to chairs can be wrongly used as restrainers.

Beds

Safety sides are often used unnecessarily and the numbers used may be related more to the attitude of the nurse in charge of the particular ward area rather than the patients' needs. Confused patients can be placed in greater danger by the use of full-length safety sides (sometimes tied on with bandages) because if they are determined to get out of bed they will fall even further when clambering over the top.

Lockers

Lockers can be wrongly positioned so that patients' independence is discouraged by their inability to deal with their personal belongings themselves.

Toileting

Too many patients are still forced to use a bedpan when, with varying degrees of independence, toileting on the lavatory or with a commode is possible.

Clothes

Dresses are sometimes put on over night clothes. Rehabilitation is actively discouraged if men attempting to walk have to hold up their ill-fitting trousers because no braces have been provided. Patients are sometimes issued with socks and stockings that do not match and which have holes in them. These practices should never happen.

One physician in geriatric medicine has suggested that those patients who on arrival in a unit are ready for immediate mobilisation (excluding the elderly seriously ill) should be assessed initially by the team and kitted out as if entering the Armed Forces, with a suitable bed, chair, locker and overbed table, as well as suitable clothes until their own can be brought in. Regular reassessment will be needed as the patient improves or deteriorates, but adequate storage space is essential for this policy to work. These suggestions may appear authoritarian, but their implementation may in the end result in more independence for the patient being rehabilitated and more happiness for the patient who has unfortunately to remain permanently in hospital.

Notes

Enquiries regarding details of specific items of equipment may be made to the authors.

1. This DHSS document is much more than a 'Building Note' as it gives excellent advice concerning the management of geriatric departments and should be consulted.

References

Agate, J.N. (1969). 'Colour in hospitals'. *World Medicine*, 4, 17, 13

Andrews, J. (1969). 'Variable-height examination couch'. *Lancet*, 2, 1231

Andrews, J. (1970). 'Geriatric ward equipment'. *British Journal of Hospital Medicine*, Equipment Supplement, April, 21

Andrews, J. (1971a). 'Hospital beds'. *Lancet*, 1, 442

Andrews, J. (1971b). 'Helping handicapped patients to have a comfortable bath'. *World Medicine*, 6, 88

Andrews, J. and Atkinson, L. (1975). 'Ward furniture and equipment in geriatric departments'. *Hospital Equipment and Supplies*, 13, 29

Andrews, J. and Atkinson, L. (1977). 'Home aids for the disabled'. *General Practitioner*, 1 July, 22

Andrews, J. and Atkinson, L. (1977/8). 'The selection of hospital equipment for use in departments of geriatric medicine'. The Association of National Health Supplies Officers

Andrews, J. and Atkinson, L. (1978). 'Selecting equipment for elderly patients in hospital'. *British Medical Journal*, 2, 484

Atkinson, L. (1971). 'Geriatric ward equipment used for assessment and re-training'. *Occupational Therapy*, 1, 442

Bliss, M.R. (1978). 'The use of ripple beds'. *Age and Ageing*, 7, 25-7

Bramwell-Jones, S. (1968). 'The needs of the disabled. A guide to the selection of household furniture'. *British Hospital Journal and Social Service Review*, LXXVII, 4058, 155

British Geriatrics Society and Royal College of Nursing Working Party (1975). *Improving Geriatric Care in Hospital.* Royal College of Nursing, London

Department of Health and Social Security (1972). *Minimum Standards in Geriatric Hospitals.* DS/72, London

Department of Health and Social Security (1977). *Domestic Services Management Advice Notes*, No. 3. General Guide to the Management of Domestic Services in the National Health Service, London

Department of Health and Social Security (1978). *Handbook of Wheelchairs and Hand-Propelled Tricycles.* Ministry of Health, 48, London

Department of Health and Social Security (1979). *Personal Handbook*, MHL 27, London

Department of Health and Social Security (1980). *Health Building Note*, No. 37

Disabled Living Foundation (1980). Information and Lists of Aids Centres in the United Kingdom. 346 Kensington High Street, London W14 8NS

Gainsborough, H. (1967). 'My second best bed'. *British Hospital Journal and Social Service Review*, 77, 859

Goldsmith, S. (1976). *Designing for the Disabled*. RIBA Publications, 3rd edition

Health Advisory Service (1977). Annual Report

Henderson, R.L. (1981). 'A new aid to geriatric nursing'. *Nursing Times*, 77

Hinchcliffe, D.J. (1980). *A patient's personalised clothing system*, Working Paper No. 27. Health Services Management Unit, Department of Social Administration, University of Manchester

Hospital Advisory Service (1969/70). Annual Report

Hospital Advisory Service (1976). Annual Report

King's Fund Working Party (1967). *Design of Hospital Bedsteads*. London

Research Institute into Consumer Affairs Comparative Test Report No. 11 (1972). *Bed/chair tables*. National Fund into Crippling Diseases. Vincent House, Springfield Road, Horsham, West Sussex RH12 1PN

Royal College of Nursing (1979). *Avoiding Low Back Injury among Nurses*

Shaw, B.H. (1979). *Mattress Coverings and their Effect on Tissue Bearing Pressures*. Biomechanical Research and Development Unit, Roehampton

Tarling, C. (1980). *Hoists and their Use*. Heinemann, for the Disabled Living Foundation, London

7 THE EFFICIENCY AND QUALITY OF THE SERVICE

E. Woodford-Williams

Many factors determine the efficiency of a geriatric department and the quality of life of the patients admitted. Simple guidelines which should enable the geriatrician to assess these aspects in his unit are outlined in this chapter. If the service is to operate successfully there must be a regular wide-ranging review of its performance.

Unit Efficiency

A great deal can be learned about the quality and standard of performance of a hospital from statistics. Unfortunately many departments of geriatric medicine fail to keep adequate statistics of their activity. As a result it is difficult to assess the workload and therefore to plan. There is almost universal failure to use the services of the Hospital Activity Analysis (HIPE). The tables in these documents show trends in different departments over several years (Statistics and Research Division, DHSS, published yearly). When reviewing and monitoring local services it is helpful to be able to compare the department's activity with that of similar departments.

A great deal can be learnt from figures showing the number of admissions, discharges and deaths over a period of years. Any changes in these figures should be investigated to identify the cause. Often it is due to a change of important staff leading to a reduction in the degree of efficiency. It is also possible to tell whether a unit is functioning well by looking at the ratio of admissions to deaths. This should arouse suspicion if the percentage of deaths related to admissions is around 35 per cent.

The yearly figures of admissions, discharges and deaths will indicate whether one is building up long-stay cases. Monitoring figures from the acute area of the unit are also valuable in this respect. In my own experience I found that if there were more than 5 people assessed as possible long-term subjects in the acute area at the end of the month in a department of 300 beds, a detailed review was indicated. This type of monthly check is a step towards improving efficiency.

The turnover of the beds is another useful indicator of performance. A unit turning over less than 5 patients per bed per year needs to be reviewed. A long waiting list of elderly patients on other wards such as orthopaedic, general medical and surgical wards is a situation which also needs examination. If the bed occupancy is high in the geriatric unit but low in the other wards consideration should be given to some re-distribution of the resources in favour of the geriatric department.

When the throughput is low on the geriatric unit, consideration should be given to staffing levels and working conditions in the wards. When staffing levels fall, consultation and communication between members decline. Nurses take short cuts and do things for patients which they could well do for themselves and patients rapidly become institutionalised. If the medical staffing is inadequate, admission and discharge procedures become haphazard and therapeutic measures are less fully discussed. Overall efficiency declines and when this occurs it is often better to reduce the number of beds to improve morale. Revans (1964) in his study on nurse management showed clearly that to overstress the staff reduces morale, increases the turnover of staff due to sickness, increases the length of stay of patients and is generally associated with inefficiency in treatment.

The acquisition of good statistical information demands a well set up office in the geriatric department, headed by a senior clerical officer and supported by at least two typists. There should also be a unit administrator for the geriatric service who would be involved in communicating and liaising with community services, the day hospital and transport. He should be part of the team and not have duties which take him away from the department, although if psychogeriatrics is integrated with the geriatric service this field of caring for the old should also be included in his job description.

The Quality of Life

Emphasis has already been placed on the importance of adequate staff levels in maintaining department efficiency. Similarly the quality of life of patients on the wards is very closely related to staffing levels. Staff shortages lead to custodial care rather than rehabilitation and most therapists consider that the key person in the rehabilitation team is the nurse. Physiotherapists, occupational therapists and speech therapists have particular skills in the assessment of need and in the techniques they use to re-educate purposeful function. Unless there are nurses in sufficient numbers and with sufficient understanding of the aims of treatment, they may well dissipate the efforts of the therapists and patients.

Sometimes it is a matter of ignorance of the importance of rehabilitation, usually it is a matter of expediency. Allowing patients to exercise the independence they have so slowly and painfully gained is inevitably time consuming and nurses have inordinate demands on their time. The use of therapy helpers to supplement the work of nurses can be invaluable, particularly in encouraging time consuming and repetitive activities and in providing physical and mental stimulus. It is axiomatic for effective rehabilitation that there is the closest collaboration between therapists and nurses to provide a consistent programme in daily living activities.

The general aim of rehabilitation should be to return the patient to familiar surroundings in the community. During the stages of treatment, therefore, contact with the patient's home and local community must be maintained and the quality of his/her life in an institutional setting considered so as to preserve his/her self image. Special care is needed to ensure that personal possessions such as clothing, glasses, hearing aids and false teeth are readily available to the patient. Of equal importance is the opportunity for patients to make decisions and manage their own affairs. Role flexibility should be fostered and patients should be encouraged to undertake and engage in roles other than 'the patient role' to prevent institutionalisation. Social and personal skills should be promoted in an active and purposeful daily programme, providing incentives which meet the emotional and physiological needs of this age group.

The quality of life in some of our hospitals has been a cause for concern and much is being done by the Department of Health and the British Geriatrics Society to improve the situation. A recent study of residential homes in London revealed staff shortages so great that only basic care of a custodial nature was possible (DHSS, 1979). Recommendations were made that residents should be encouraged to maintain their own sense of personal worth and self respect and that those concerned should appraise the quality of life of residents with a view to helping them maintain links with the past, to enjoy the present and to have confidence in the future. Only a few of the officers in the homes considered their task might include a rehabilitative aspect. A significant number were against encouraging it!

The Health Advisory Service

An important step in improving the efficiency and quality of the service for the elderly was the establishment of the Hospital Advisory Service (HAS) in 1969 by Richard Crossman, the Secretary of State for Social Services. The aim was to help improve the management of patient care in individual hospitals and to advise the Secretaries of State about conditions in hospitals in England and Wales. Factors leading to the decision to set up this body are described in the Annual Report of the Department of Health and Social Security for 1969. Details of the mode of initial operation are described in the first of 7 annual reports of the Hospital Advisory Service (1971). The remit was altered in 1976 and the name was changed to the Health Advisory Service. Emphasis since then has concentrated on the development of constructive attitudes and relationships and on the promotion of effective co-ordination of health and complementary local authority services. The aim has been to propagate good ideas and practice and to encourage local solutions to local problems.

Although the HAS operates independently of the Department of Health and Social Security and the Welsh Office, it can make information available to these departments about the hospitals and community services with which it has been involved. As an advisory body it does not investigate individual complaints. Multidisciplinary teams visit hospitals and look at the full range of services and consider how they conform to the norms and minimum standards and the policies set regionally or nationally. In particular, information is sought and advice given on:

1. The service the hospital affords the community and the links it has with the community.
2. Relations between the staff and patients.
3. The physical conditions and staff ratios within the hospital.
4. The operational policies and performance of the unit.

In general, hospital staff welcome the opportunity of discussing their services with fellow professionals and welcome the opportunities of looking critically at the various alternatives available. Too often, hospitals labour under difficulties and are frequently reluctant to face unpleasant solutions, particularly those created by faulty organisation, lack of resources and personality problems. Over the years it has become apparent that the HAS is important in facilitating change, and in particular in promoting multidisciplinary teamwork.

Prior to visits by the HAS notices are posted in hospitals inviting comments on the services provided and letters are also sent to recently discharged patients and their relatives. A study of the comments made reveals that most are appreciative of the services given and they relate deficiencies to staff shortages. On the negative side, mention is made of the lack of communication between doctors and patients. Many would like to know more about their illness and treatment. People also resent being placed in wards with patients with whom they cannot communicate. They describe the waste of food in hospitals and the lack of services at night.

Among the units visited by the HAS were a number providing a very high standard of practice. Indeed some units could be regarded as models in certain aspects of care, for example, in acute, rehabilitation or long-term care, but it is perhaps significant to note that all units providing a better service had most of the following features:

1. At least one-third and sometimes one-half or more of the total allocation of geriatric beds were in a district hospital where full pathological, X-ray and other services were available. The remaining beds were usually in peripheral units. The total number of beds in most departments corresponded with the national norm of 10 per 1,000 population over 65 years but others were more often below than above this.

2. Although buildings were seldom new, there had been imaginative up-grading. The wards were not overcrowded. Adequate privacy had been provided for patients and there was easy access to a sufficient number of toilets. There were separate areas for the alert and for the confused patients. The equipment on the ward was of good standard and therapists were usually involved in decisions as to the best use and choice of equipment.

3. Successful units gave more attention to the content of the patients' day. There was more participation of nursing staff with therapists in rehabilitating patients and the incontinence rate was low. Few cot sides and restricting chairs were used and the participation rate of patients was high in the activities of daily living.

4. Practices such as 'intermittent admission', holiday relief and progressive patient care were followed. The geriatric department had usually made a commitment *to provide a comprehensive in-patient and outpatient service, accepting the care of all patients*

referred to them by general practitioners on an age-related basis.
Patients needing urgent admission were sent directly to the unit
so that the department was able *to deal with their problem from
the start.* This provides a more effective use of beds than allowing
a patient to linger in an acute medical ward awaiting transfer to
the geriatric wards. *A significantly high proportion of new outpatients were seen in the better units* and some of the more
progressive held at least one clinic a day. Clinics were held either
at the hospitals, or in the day hospital or in health centres.
Efficient outpatient services ensured that there were always beds
available for patients who really needed them. Where adequate
outpatient services existed the waiting list was minimal.

5. The participation of trained social workers *before the patient's
admission or immediately after was very important* so that help
could be offered to the family as quickly as possible. In this way
integration and resettlement into the community was far more
successful than when family difficulties were not properly understood until the patient was ready for discharge. At that stage it is
often too late. Social workers and occupational therapists also
made domiciliary visits so that the whole picture was available.
Domiciliary visits were also made by some consultants to prevent
inappropriate admissions but the more outpatient work done the
fewer domiciliary visits by doctors were necessary.

6. In successful departments emphasis was placed on both multidisciplinary management and clinical conferences. A number of
units had a health visitor/community nurse attached to them and
she acted in liaison with colleagues in the community and visited
patients at home after discharge. Good relations also existed
between the consultants in geriatric medicine and their colleagues
in other departments such as psychiatry and orthopaedic surgery.
Usually there was also *good collaboration between the department and outside bodies such as local authorities, social services,
housing departments and voluntary bodies.*

7. It was usual to find that the administrative staff of the hospital
had favourable attitudes towards the geriatric department.
Medical records were better kept and some had adopted the
'Weed' system (Weed, 1971). An information booklet listing
services available was a feature of some units as well as written procedures for admissions, discharges, deaths and prescriptions, etc. It
is significant that good units had a better than average establishment
of clerical and secretarial help and they produced an annual

report on the activity of the unit.

8. Units providing a good service also had a higher than average establishment of medical staff but fewer beds than average. As well as more than one consultant, these units frequently had junior staff in training grades such as registrars and general practitioner trainees. Rotation of staff with other branches of medicine was encouraged. Most of the units had active training programmes for their staff but regrettably, owing to lack of facilities and time, few were able to undertake research.

The evidence suggests that the quality of a unit depends very much on the quality of the multidisciplinary team and in particular on its leadership. Even with the best physical conditions and facilities the milieu will not necessarily improve unless there is good leadership. 'No battle was lost until its leader thought it so' (Earl Haig).

The aged are an underprivileged group in the community today. It is our duty to assess and cater for their needs, to train staff and stimulate research in all aspects of ageing. This demands efficient use of scarce resources if all those who need help are to get it without delay. The task is daunting, but in no other field of medicine are the skills of nurses, doctors, therapists and others needed more by patients, their relatives and the state.

References

Department of Health and Social Security (1969). Annual Report. HMSO, London

Department of Health and Social Security (1979). *Residential Care for the Elderly in London*. A study by the DHSS Social Work Service, London

National Health Service annual Report of the Hospital Advisory Service to the Secretary of State for Social Services and the Secretary of State for Wales for Year 1969-1970. HMSO, London (1971). Ibid for years 1971 (1972), 1972 (1973), 1973 (1974), 1974 (1975), 1975 (1976), 1976 (1977)

Revans, R.W. (1964). *Standards of Morale*. Oxford University Press, London

Weed, L.L. (1971). *Medical Records, Medical Education and Patient Care*. Year Book Medical Publishers, Chicago

ATTITUDES, TEAMWORK, CO-ORDINATION
AND COMMUNICATION

J.T. Leeming

If you have recently been appointed a Consultant Physician in geriatric
medicine, the development of the care of the elderly in your district
will henceforth depend in large measure on your leadership. Your role
will have two main functions, medicine and management. As a doctor,
you will be expected to provide health care for older people with acute
and longer-term illness and disability, and to give advice to general
practitioners, your hospital colleagues and others. As a manager, you
will need to set up and maintain a service framework in which health
care can be carried out to the highest standard, and you will have to
build harmonious relationships with all relevant staff in hospital and
community. No matter how busy you are it is important that you keep
a good proportion of your time and energy for each of these functions.

There is no single ideal way to run a department. In addition to your
knowledge and experience of what has been done elsewhere you will
have to take into account local assets and restraints in both buildings
and staff, and your decisions will also be influenced by your own
personality and interests. My purpose is more to help you to ask the
right questions than to give the answers.

Attitudes and teamwork are considered first because these emotive
and somewhat nebulous concepts are often thought of as the most
important influences for good or ill on the success of a department.
However, you may well derive more benefit from devoting energy to
establishing good practices in the less emotive and more clear-cut areas
of co-ordination and communication and these are discussed in the
second half of the chapter.

Attitudes

If you think that a member of staff is a 'dead loss', do you tell him so?
Probably not. Do you, however, say as much to your close colleagues
whom you meet frequently and get on well with? It is quite probable
that you do. Whatever you say, you are unlikely to discuss your
difficult problems with such a person, and in such dealings as you have

with him you may well betray a lack of confidence in his judgement. Your junior staff are likely to share your attitude but may mask it less effectively. It is easy to see that such negative attitudes can be very disturbing for the person to whom they relate. Those concerned tend to drift apart. Ignorance of each other's assets then grows, and what may have started from pure misunderstanding can become a serious 'personality' problem. Situations like this can arise all too quickly, for we all tend to develop, on the basis of a small number of unhappy experiences, stereotypes of people that we 'can't stand' and, if the object of our disapproval fits one of these patterns, he may be relegated to the 'dead loss' category almost on sight.

Attitudes cannot be directly observed, they are infectious, and they are as much affected by past events and personalities as by facts about the person or situation to which they relate. They set in train a sequence of behaviour which makes them self-fulfilling. They tend to be mutually reinforcing. Thus, if you harbour a negative attitude for a long period towards somebody (e.g. 'hate his guts'), then it is likely that he will come to feel similarly about you. It is important to realise that when somebody does not do what you would like him to do, it does not necessarily indicate a negative attitude. He may disagree, he may have had second thoughts, he may have forgotten, he may not have received your message, he may have had to do something else urgently, he may have been unwell, and so on.

What should you do about negative attitudes in others? Don't take it personally or emotionally for little can be done when these things become a matter of warring personalities and emotional conflicts. The dire situation which can arise is starkly stated by Brill (1976) who observes that when a person perceives another person as a threat to his identity and rights, a bitter struggle may ensue in which

> reality orientation may be lost, and the opposition may be endowed with qualities of evil that can only be dealt with by total destruction. An atmosphere of mistrust, fear, and hatred may develop that makes constructive use of this kind of conflict difficult. There is a tendency to personalise the situation that not only intensifies the feelings involved but also makes constructive resolution difficult.

Even though it does you good to 'have a good grumble', do not over-indulge in your own dislikes and other negative attitudes, either in your own thoughts or in discussion with staff and colleagues and do not make hasty judgements. Remember that attitudes cannot be changed overnight.

Do make sure that your own house is in order, for this will result in your merit being recognised in due course. Review your approach from time to time. Are your own attitudes positive enough? Are you giving your own staff enough support and encouragement? Take opportunities to get to know your colleagues better, and show an interest in their work, aspirations and problems, rather than just parading your own. Ask yourself whether your department adequately reflects active policies and an optimistic philosophy. As Millard (1976) puts it, have you developed 'a service that is not geared to perceived ideas [attitudes?] of people, but tailored to the needs of the individual patient, taking into account the medical diagnosis, social diagnosis, prognosis for life, and the expectations of each patient?' Your department should reflect an enthusiasm for all the good things about being old, rather than a losing battle against physical and mental decay. This is the stance that will convince sceptics that you are working on the right lines.

Teamwork

There is general agreement that many professions need to work together in geriatric medicine because of the complex factors that contribute to illness and disability at this stage in life, and which may need consideration in depth during diagnosis and treatment (see Figure 8.1).

Figure 8.1: The Complex Situation of the Ill Older Person

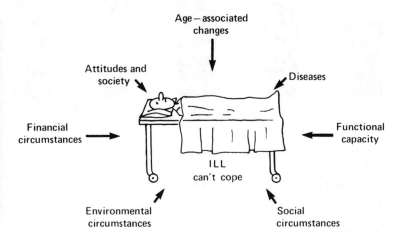

Geriatricians are well aware of the need for a good multidisciplinary team. Who, then, is in this team, and what is the relative importance of each member? Will the same team apply to all situations, and will the importance of each member vary? Let us define the team as 'those who are necessary for successful diagnosis and treatment'. Before you read on, may I suggest that you consider those that you would include in the team in three different situations, and that you sketch a bar chart with a bar for each team member, the height of the bar representing his relative importance. The three situations are

1. The team for your normal daily work.
2. Specifically, the team for a patient admitted with a chest infection and melaena.
3. The team for a patient who needs rehabilitation following a colostomy.

Your first team may include the staff shown in Figure 8.2. It would

Figure 8.2: Team for Normal Daily Work

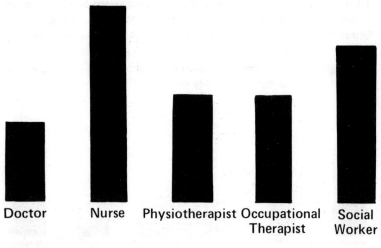

be surprising if the height of your bars did not accord the doctor more importance than I have shown in the figure. But suppose we were considering quality of care? In that case the nurse would tend to have a more important role, showing that the relative importance of staff varies with the task under consideration. What would the speech therapist have to say about this illustration?

For the patient with a chest infection and melaena, the team might be as in Figure 8.3. The diagnosis could not be made without the help of

Figure 8.3: Team for Patient with Chest Infection and Melaena

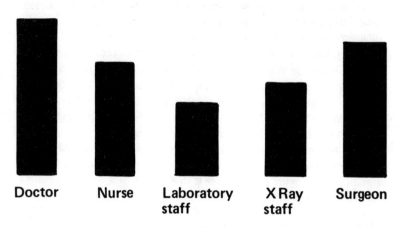

laboratory and X-ray staff and a surgeon may be essential for treatment.

Our patient with a colostomy may require the services of the staff shown in Figure 8.4. If there is a stoma therapist in the district, she

Figure 8.4: Team for Patient Requiring Rehabilitation following a Colostomy

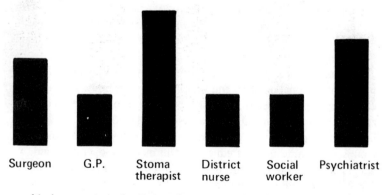

would play a major role. Quite a large proportion of patients who have a colostomy develop depression and may need help from a psychiatrist. Some of these patients may have inadequate toilet facilities at home and may need assistance from the social worker for rehousing. Others may have problems of manual dexterity for which the additional help of a physiotherapist and an occupational therapist might have to be requested.

Thus the team, and the relative significance of each member, varies according to the patient's condition and according to the task we select. In either case, relative inputs may be perceived differently by different members of the team.

Why is it that we consider teamwork to be more significant in geriatric medicine than in other specialties? Perhaps it is because of the differences in the professions with whom we need to work closely, and because we need to study the patient's home situation. Perhaps we are able to take a broader, team-based approach because technology generally plays a smaller role in the treatment of our patients.

I did not include the patient and his relatives in the team. Should I have done so? After all, they are the only factor common to all three situations (see Figure 8.5). It is clear that to talk of a 'team' meaning a fixed group of people is an oversimplification. It is more useful to consider those who need to work together in each case, and 'working together' is a more accurate description of the process than 'teamwork'.

When staff of different professions work together misunderstandings and loss of efficiency can occur and these may relate to, for example, professional roles, personalities, the length of time staff have worked together, the need for some overlapping of roles, professional rivalry, hierarchical structures, and differences in the number of staff in different professions.

Staff function both as representatives of a profession with a specific training programme and ladder of promotion (see Figure 8.6) and as individuals with their own unique personalities and family backgrounds (see Figure 8.7).

Performance may be enhanced or limited by whether a task fits in with their personal qualities and whether it is appropriate for their career development. Staff need time, both to get to know each other as individuals and as members of different professions, and to work out how best to contribute to the task in hand. In many multidisciplinary groups, staff come and go frequently. This makes co-operation and understanding more difficult, but also prevents the group becoming fossilised and rigid in its approach.

Given the complexity of patients' needs and problems, and the number of staff involved, the planning and co-ordination of treatment is a skilled task. There needs to be a common core of knowledge, and a willingness to accept some overlapping of roles so that those who are

Figure 8.5: Additional Members of the Team?

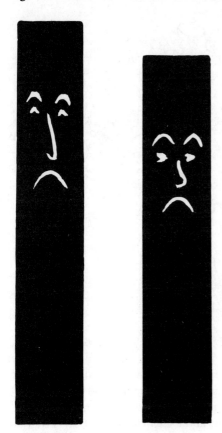

Patient   Relatives

doing most of the work in a particular case can play a key role without
overlooking factors which, strictly speaking, come within the province
of another profession. Overlapping of roles should occur, for example,
between nurses and therapists with regard to enabling patients to dress
and walk. It will not be necessary for a therapist to be involved in every
case. The nurse then takes the role of key worker. Not infrequently,
when the concepts of overlapping roles or key workers are first suggested,
it is seen as an attempt at unwarranted encroachment by one or more
professions on the cherished territory of others (see Figure 8.8).

The levels of hierarchy, when their incumbents are not included in

Figure 8.6: The Team as Professionals

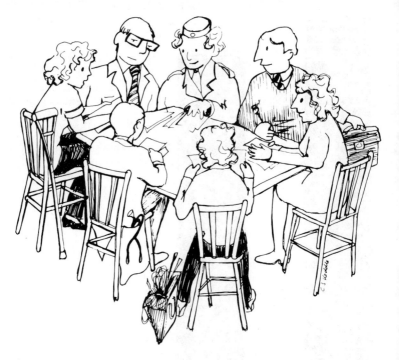

the day-to-day team, constitute another cherished territory which must receive due recognition and respect. A good team is a fertile source of new ideas and suggestions, but these cannot be implemented without the active support of senior staff in the discipline concerned. A clinical team must have a mechanism for discussion with such staff, who may otherwise be justifiably disconcerted by events and react against new practices. A word at the right time can save much unnecessary anguish.

The factor of differences in numbers of staff of different professions is especially relevant with regard to nurses who make up by far the largest group. In hospital there might be, for instance, 150 nurses, 20 domestic staff, 10 porters, 4 doctors, 4 physiotherapists, 2 occupational therapists, 1 or 2 social workers and 1 speech therapist. The large number of nursing staff is not always given enough weight as a potential cause of misunderstanding, which can occur on both sides. On the one hand, if there is a representative from each profession on a team then there is a risk that the nurses will feel that due weight is not being given to their point of view. If, on the other hand, there is proportional representation,

Figure 8.7: The Team as Individuals

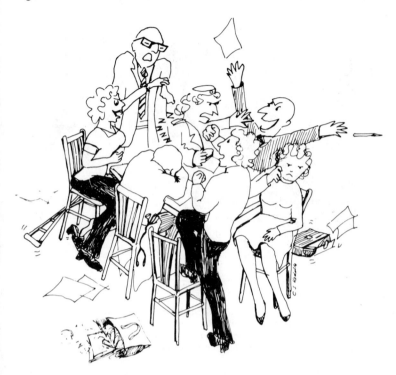

the other professions may feel dominated by nurses. Nurse management varies in the efficiency with which information is distributed
within its ranks, and other professionals vary in their readiness to
appreciate the nursing point of view.

In working closely together some conflict is inevitable. It is important
that all concerned should recognise this as a normal and healthy human
characteristic to be handled with understanding and good humour. Otherwise the group will fall apart or duck important issues to avoid conflict.
Such avoidance of contentious issues in order to avoid unpleasantness
was found to occur between health visitors and general practitioners by
Gilmore *et al.* (1974). Two kinds of conflict occur. The first is the
more heated variety which I have already described, relating to such
matters as incompatible attitudes, professional status and territory, and
the second is straightforward honest disagreement about day-to-day
judgements and decisions. Often both kinds of conflict happen at the
same time. The production of destructive levels of heat from the first

Figure 8.8: Professional Territories

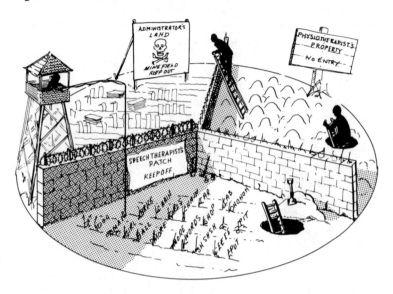

I am grateful to Ken Etherington, of the Visual Aids Department, Newcastle Poly-
technic, for permission to use Figure 8.8 re-drawn from his illustration in *Working
Together: aspects of providing a multi-disciplinary service for mentally handicapped
people*, 1979, Association of Professions for the Mentally Handicapped, London

kind can be prevented or minimised by understanding the types of difficulty
which commonly arise, some of which I have outlined. The second kind is
bound to occur in a process of constructive discussion. A team without any
conflict is in a bad way and will produce little of value. It may postpone
decisions on the grounds that consensus has not been reached.

Leadership is necessary to facilitate wise and timely decisions, to resolve
disputes on questions such as who should be involved, who does what, who
needs to be informed and to ensure that the wishes and needs of the patient,
rather than the staff, are being met. But the words 'leader' and 'leadership'
are also emotive and often misunderstood. Gross oversimplification of the
issues is usual. Disputes occur on whether there should be a leader, on who
the leader should be, and whether it should always be the same person.
Doctors may insist that 'the consultant must be the leader', and other professionals may disagree with this. Being leader is sometimes thought of as
'showing who's boss', 'starting as we mean to go on' and 'making decisions
and sticking to them'. It is said that there 'must be a strong leader' and yet

what does 'strong leader' mean in a group where success depends on each person thinking for himself and giving a considered opinion on matters in which he has special knowledge and training and, above all, interest? How should the consultant lead when he may see each patient for ten minutes or less each week, whereas the other members average some two hours and often much more? Of what relevance is 'starting as we mean to go on' when policies and goals have to be changed frequently because of changing circumstances and wide fluctuations in the fitness of patients? If we stick to decisions come hell or high water, whom does this benefit, and are there more realistic ways of achieving efficiency as measured by patient turnover and a capacity to respond to requests from the community?

Clinical teams are likely to have between four and ten members. It is advantageous if three or four of them are experienced members of the department and remain within the team for a long period. This provides stability and each can help with the leadership role. This sub-group should learn how to exploit their complementary characteristics (e.g. peacemaker, record keeper, ideas person, reference-finder, morale raiser). If there is only one experienced member it is difficult to prevent confusion and uncertainty arising, especially if he is unable to spend much time with the members between meetings.

Kane (1975) defines leadership as 'any conscious act of influence over the behaviour of others'. Clearly, this is a process in which all of us engage. It is a dynamic force which should be guided rather than limited.

What are the qualifications for leadership within a multidisciplinary team? Here are some suggestions:

A liking for people and an understanding of the way they behave in groups, both as individuals and as members of a profession.
A knowledge of the aims of the department, and of how the team concerned relates to these aims.
A willingness to listen and to welcome constructive criticism.
A strong sense of purpose and an ability to communicate this to others
A rich sense of humour.
An ability to attend meetings of the team regularly.
A good sense of time.

Should the consultant be the titular leader? If he has the qualifications I have listed, the answer is 'yes', but there is something wrong if he has to insist on it. His proper function is not so much to bang the drum (though this is necessary from time to time) as to foster leadership qualities in other members of the team. Inexperienced staff will be overawed, and need encouragement to participate. Steering a path between naive, overenthusiastic support and overbearing criticism is a skilled but very worthwhile task.

Co-ordination

For our present purpose, co-ordination means the setting up of an organisational framework, or network, which will enable those who need to communicate to do so. The framework should reflect the aims of the service and facilitate the achievement of these aims with the least amount of effort and misunderstanding. It should leave staff as free as possible to get on with their daily work, help them to reach the highest possible standard of performance, and facilitate the introduction of change when that is required.

You will find it helpful to have a number of basic questions in mind when reviewing your organisation, such as the following:

Are the needs of patients being met?
Are staff able to do their job properly?
Are the educational needs of staff being met?
Is there a need for social functions to help staff to relax, get to know each other and enjoy themselves together?
Is there a need for research to see whether the best practices are in use?
Is there adequate planning for the immediate, medium and long-term future?

These questions need consideration in relation to various levels and spheres of activity (see Table 8.1), and in relation to different groups of staff (see Table 8.2).

You should review your policies with regard to all these levels and staff groupings annually, or more frequently if necessary. Medical staff (see Table 8.2) are the group to consider first because your efforts with other professions cannot flourish to the full unless you have created a good understanding with the doctors in your area, starting with those in your department. If you are joining a team of two or more consultants, you will need to work out your relationships with them. This can then be incorporated in a departmental policy statement on how you plan to complement each other's efforts. Your own junior medical staff will need their duties defined and a good job description is useful here. Job

Table 8.1

Levels of activity	Relevant practices or committees
Delivery of care (patients and relatives)	Are patients/relatives able to see you on your own?
Wards, outpatient clinics, day hospital	Rounds, case conferences
Department of geriatric medicine as a whole	Departmental meetings
The hospital as a whole	Medical division, medical executive, meetings of heads of departments
The district	Health care planning team for the elderly, district management team

Table 8.2

Groups of staff (Hospital *and* Community)	Relevant practices or committees
Medical	
In your department	Meetings on (a) day-to-day matters, (b) education/research
Other hospital specialties	Clinical meetings, medical division
Community physicians	District management team, health care planning team for the elderly
General practitioners	Local medical committee, domiciliary visits, postgraduate meetings
Others	
Nursing and administrative	District management team, health care planning team for the elderly, heads of departments meetings, *ad hoc* meetings with individuals
Therapy	Heads of department meetings, 'Topic' discussions with whole multidisciplinary team
Social work	Heads of department meetings
Volunteers	League of Friends, or equivalent, Age Concern

descriptions are sent out to applicants and a good one attracts good applicants as well as guiding them when they start work. Your staff will need support and advice as well as scope for independent action. Remember to encourage them and help them with their careers. With regard to his own medical team Irvine (1976) observes that 'although we share an office we do not all meet at any time in the week unless we arrange to do so. We have a weekly firm meeting from 8.30 am to 9.00 am and a journal club on another morning. This ensures that we are together for at least an hour a week and provides an invaluable opportunity for us to keep in touch and to discuss the innumerable points which come up in the running of a large medical team'. Irvine also stresses the importance of good relationships with general practitioners and comments that 'the geriatric physician, like all other consultants, shares with the general practitioner the care of the patient in hospital. He meets the general practitioner on domiciliary visits, at the postgraduate centre, and at conferences in the geriatric unit. An important part of the geriatric physician's job is to know the general practitioners and to make himself available to them.'

The nursing and administrative professions are also worth special mention. Because of the clinical importance and the large number of nurses, and their hierarchical management structure, it is a good plan to meet the senior administrative nurse on a regular basis so that issues and ideas can be discussed at leisure and in confidence.

The administrator can be of immense help in getting your co-ordinative structures right, partly because this is his special area of expertise and partly because of his position in the organisation. He can be an invaluable link-person between groups and grades of staff. By his attendance at meetings, the administrator sees all professional groups and trade union representatives at first hand, and is uniquely placed to get to know their idiosyncrasies, strengths and weaknesses. Also his non-involvement in patient care means that he can approach clinical staff without any suspicion that he wishes to question their professional judgement or poach on their jealously guarded terrain.

You may find it useful to regard yourself, the senior nurse and the administrator as a 'key team'. This brings together the main types of management skill needed and makes a good base from which to communicate with all staff. It simplifies the task and, because so few people are involved, it is possible to have frequent discussions. Such key teams have been found to work well for programmes for improving geriatric care in hospital (see DHSS enclosure to HN (79)35). Even such a small group will not meet regularly by chance. A time and place must be agreed, and this will only happen if there is a common understanding of the tasks to be achieved and agreement on priorities.

Communication

The need for communication is not always easy to appreciate. When we are very preoccupied with a set of problems we tend erroneously to assume that others share our concern and knowledge. Moreover, good communication is hard work; it entails much use of our critical faculties, which tire easily. For my present purpose I will define communication as – the exchange of such messages, observations, knowledge, statements, ideas, thoughts and opinions as are necessary for your department to achieve optimal function. By definition the exchange of information is a two-way process, with a minimum of two participants. Communication is not complete unless the message has been both received and understood. Figure 8.9 summarises the processes relevant to communication, each of which will be discussed briefly.

Figure 8.9: Processes Relevant to Communication

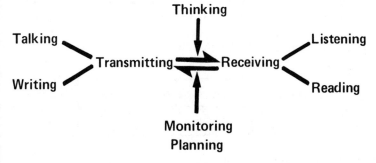

Spoken communication may be face-to-face or by telephone. Face-to-face communication can be on a one-to-one basis or in informal groups or formal meetings. It allows immediate feedback, and the reactions of others can be gauged by tone of voice and by non-verbal reactions such as expressions, posture, gesture and so on. It can only involve those present. For formal meetings a previously circulated agenda and minutes are essential. A common fault in meetings is to spend too much time discussing matters concerning people who are not present.

The telephone also allows immediate feedback, but without the non-verbal element. It saves travel time. It is important to ascertain that the recipient of your call is not in the middle of a busy meeting or clinic. The GPO can arrange for several people to be in touch at the same time for a 'telephone conference' (Leeming and Carver, 1979).

Written communication is more impersonal and takes longer, but allows for more organisation of material. If typed, it will be more legible than if handwritten, and a carbon copy can be kept as a record. Photocopies and stencilled copies are even more impersonal but can be circulated to any number of people. There are non-verbal aspects to written communication. Thus a handwritten letter may suggest a desire for confidentiality, a more friendly and personal approach, a conscientious effort to avoid delay, a lack of secretarial assistance, or just bad organisation, according to the circumstances. The use of a pocket dictating machine saves an enormous amount of secretarial time, and enables dictation to be done at any place or time, the only snag being that it becomes easy to say too much.

It is important to show an equal interest in listening to the views of others as in imparting your views to them. Good listeners are harder to find than good talkers. Listening demands mental energy and concentration, and is a much more active and complex process than is apparent to the observer. As Marson (1977) points out, in a discussion the person who is not talking is in fact engaged in many activities (see Figure 8.10). It is important to talk to people in surroundings and at

Figure 8.10: The Active Listener

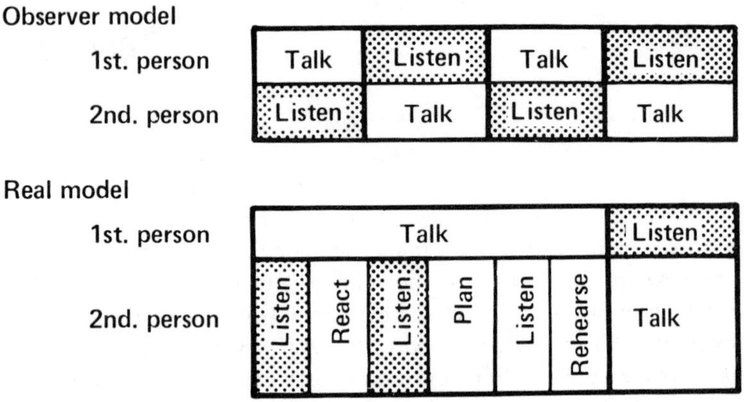

times when they can pay attention. The speaker must not overload the listener and should test whether he has been understood from time to time.

Reading is an activity in which doctors get a great deal of practice, and yet, how much of what we read through each week do we really digest? How much potentially interesting material do we skip? May I suggest that you re-read and analyse in detail a medical article that you have read recently? As you read note down your answers to the following questions:

1. What is the purpose of the article?
2. How does it go about achieving its purpose?
3. Is the evidence clearly presented?
4. What questions would you like to ask the author if you were attempting to repeat his work?
5. Do you consider the conclusions proven?
6. Are there any unjustified speculations made?

To answer all these questions may take some considerable time but you will almost certainly view the article in a new light when you have finished. Obviously, there is not time to read everything in such detail, but the conclusion to be drawn is clear. Do not accept what you read without critical analysis, do not overestimate the amount you can read thoroughly, and set aside adequate time for the systematic appraisal of important documents or articles. Be sure that your writing is brief and to the point. Set it out clearly and logically and give evidence for any assertions made.

Keep your readership in mind whilst you are writing. It is often impossible to write material which will be equally acceptable and accessible to all those you wish to inform, and you may need to produce two or more versions.

Thinking, planning and monitoring are three essential catalysts for good communication. Think before you speak—how often have we heard that remark, and how often failed to comply? It is not easy to get it right all the time. Sometimes a timely loss of temper can be invaluable. Letters written in a foul temper are usually better torn up and reconsidered, so make sure that you see them before they are sent out. Think what you really want to say or write and why. Is now the right time or place? Are there better ways of achieving the same end? Do you need more information? Have you met the people concerned? If not, then it may be best to go and see them, or ask them to come and see you. The quality of communication improves greatly when the participants have met and know each other. In many cases a mixture of written and spoken communication is best; for example it is a good plan to follow up a lunchtime chat or phone call with a memo summarising what was said and the action proposed. To achieve a high take-up rate with a large number of people use a number of channels, such as word of mouth, letters to key individuals, newsletters and notice boards. You have to select the right channels for your purpose.

Monitor your communication systems from time to time. Are you putting out up-to-date information? Do you need to revise job descriptions, patient information booklets, guidelines for procedures or referral forms? What (if anything) goes wrong and why? Are general practitioners and others satisfied with the information they receive when patients return home? Are there aspects about which they would like to know more? Do night staff know what goes on in the daytime? Do the day staff have any difficulties getting information from each other? Is there unnecessary duplication of effort? How do staff of the many professions concerned get the information they need to do their job? In other words, what are the lines of communication? Who are the key communicators in your department? If the ward clerk is the only person present on the ward every day of the week, is her potential for helping communications being adequately realised?

In your management role you will need to ask questions like these frequently. How else could you elicit the information you need? Most staff prefer to be asked how things are going than to be given orders. Management has much to do with the art of asking the right questions. I have indicated, in a structured and perhaps rather academic manner, some of the major directions that your enquiries could usefully take. A structured, logical approach is of great value, but do not let this lead you to neglect the promptings of intuition or inspiration. You may find wise counsellors quite outside the boundaries I have drawn, and many of your best ideas may come to you in the bath.

References

Brill, N.I. (1976). *Teamwork: Working Together in the Human Services.* J.B. Lippincott, Philadelphia

DHSS (1978). Enclosure to HN(79)35, December. 'A programme for improving geriatric care in hospital.' Report of a working group.

Gilmore, M., Bruce, N. and Hunt, M. (1974). *The Work of the Nursing Team in General Practice.* Council for the Education and Training of Health Visitors, London

Irvine, R.E. (1976). 'Teamwork, Links with other Specialties and Community Services', in *Doctors and Old Age*, J.T. Leeming (ed.), British Geriatrics Society, Mitcham

Kane, R.A. (1975). 'The interprofessional team as a small group', *Social Work in Health Care*, I, 19-32

Leeming, J.T. and Carver, V. (1979). 'Working together', Unit 14 of course P252. 'An ageing population', Open University Press, Milton Keynes

Marson, S.N. (1977). *Working with People, an Interactive Approach.* NHS Learning

Resources Unit, Sheffield
Millard, P.H. (1976). 'Attitudes and Geriatrics', in *Doctors and Old Age*, J.T.
Leeming (ed.). British Geriatrics Society, Mitcham

9 COMMUNITY SERVICES FOR THE ELDERLY

G. Schroeder and D. Coakley

Most governments take a certain degree of responsibility for the provision of health care services for the elderly and there is a prevalent view today that offering supportive care at home is preferable to uprooting old people and sending them into institutions. Local arrangements for the provision of care will depend on the policy of individual states or countries. The history of local institutions and patterns of care must therefore be understood when developing a geriatric service.

A list of community support services can only suggest what people need in the home to strengthen domestic care and to prevent institutionalisation. The descriptive list of practical requirements in this chapter attempts to bear in mind two different systems of health care planning. The community care planning of the UK represents a government's attempt to provide and maintain, in part through its statutes, a very comprehensive human service to a vulnerable sector of the population. In the USA, states have traditionally preferred less centralisation of power. The federal government has a narrower brief. It takes fiscal and national policy decisions but the details and the scope of health programmes are determined at local level and carried out by both state and voluntary bodies, often predominantly the latter.

The National Health Service in the UK has addressed itself to a very wide area of need in health care. It works in close administrative conjunction with the social services, which have quite comprehensive responsibilities in issues of family life.

The following analysis of useful support services is based on the pattern used in local authority in the UK, rather than on systems obtaining in the USA, because the British government's more broadly-based concept of need includes those grey areas which cannot easily be defined within the limits of finance or health, but which often become the central issues in care for the elderly. This choice is not to belittle the sizeable presence and vital contribution in England of the voluntary agencies, whose practical planning and services have long formed the basis of community care.

The history of the Jewish Board of Guardians in the UK provides a fascinating and instructive account of a voluntary agency's growth and flexible adaptation to changing needs and finally to the establishment of

132

the Welfare State whose territory covered so much that previously had been the concern of the voluntary organisations alone (Lipman, 1959). Age Concern is a voluntary organisation which has promoted the welfare of Britain's elderly over the past 40 years. Today it is actively involved in practical programmes, information services, national campaigning, training programmes and research projects. It has a publications section which is invaluable to anyone involved in services for the elderly (Age Concern, 1980).

When there is no national health service, as for example in the USA, the patterns of community care follow the historical development of the voluntary organisations. Until recently, apart from the Social Security Act which reflected primarily a concern with financial provision, federal legislation has been limited to the Medicare programme (a health insurance entitlement to those of pensionable age).

Considerable local variation exists in service areas that come under the umbrella of Medicaid (aid for health-related expenses), the state discretionary programme grant-aided by the federal government. Here a means test determines eligibility, services are not necessarily time-limited as in Medicare, and some social services are added to the medical/health-related ones (Davidson and Marmor, 1980). Every state now must maintain an Office for the Ageing and information on the network of local services should be available there. These would include the state programmes operating under Medicaid as well as the services offered by local voluntary organisations and local branches of national groups such as the National Retired Teachers Association/American Association of Retired Persons, which is an active agency in the service of the elderly.

The variety of potential community support services in any area in the USA will depend upon the sophistication of local voluntary agencies and citizen groups in the matter of writing proposals to qualify for federal funding under titles of the Older Americans Act of 1965. Many imaginative and sensitively conceived services may exist in an area, but they may be ephemeral if they were originally funded as demonstration programmes, subsequently failing to get any permanent status after their trial run. It is here that a geriatric unit may have a contribution to make in substantiating need.

It is important to ensure continuity. Whereas in the UK there are two state bodies with a mandate to maintain basic services (the area health authorities and the social service departments), in the USA there is no obligation on the part of state or federal bodies to ensure continuity of services which may have originated in the voluntary sector in response to a need.

The larger organisations will be likely to be more secure, since they will have fund-raising and fund-maintaining expertise as part of their make-up. It is the smaller, 'grass-roots' enterprises that are at risk, such as a single luncheon club or a peripatetic large-print book service, which may die for lack of funds with the expiry of a federal grant. In this context, good communication, which is one of the mainstays of effective community care, cannot be neglected. Hospitals should take an active interest in the fate of the supportive services they hope to make use of, because any that have not gained security under the hospital follow-up entitlements of Medicare or the supplementary health finance of Medicaid are not guaranteed continued existence.

The supportive aftercare services which the community may offer should reinforce the life of the patient in many areas outside the formal territory of health care. It is worth looking in some detail at the actual manpower needs of a person who is taking up the threads of his life again after discharge from a geriatric unit. He wants security of food and shelter and above all the chance to continue being the person he is in the place that he came from. The fabric of social and medical support that keeps a pensioner at home must be understood in terms of these basic needs.

The range of community services detailed in this chapter is suggested by the maximum help that someone may need. In fact many elderly people can get most of what they require from their family or friends. For those who are less fortunate in human and financial resources the same need for continuity of life style and a sense of personal independence exists, and it is this independence which is the key consideration in aftercare provision. Physical handicap may need to be compensated for by extra human aid or mechanical devices; social life may need active stimulation; and the ability to maintain independence may have to be consciously preserved. If once an elderly person is made to feel that the struggle for independence and self-determination is hopeless, then he is likely to choose unnecessary institutional care, or a passive role at home which makes heavy demands on those who care for him.

Much of the help and technical equipment which someone may need in order to manage after discharge from hospital is centred around the home and its daily running. Where the household already contains family or friends, less outside help may be required. The ways in which a geriatric unit can help support this primary and vital caring unit, the family, will be examined later. For the elderly frail couple or single person, domestic supplements are likely to be needed. It is, however, the greatest mistake to imagine that even the most ingenious and well-manned auxiliary force will guarantee successful discharge if the individual character and preferences of the patient have been overlooked. Planning starts with the person.

Home Help or Homemaker Service

A home help is someone who supplements the strength of frail house-keepers. The service generally involves 1-3 hours per day for a number of days per week depending on individual need. The usual tasks performed are household cleaning, tidying, bed-making, sometimes meal preparation, shopping or escorting to shops, pension-collection, and a multitude of general small errands. A home help extends the physical abilities of a handicapped or frail person thus helping to keep the household running. Escorting an elderly person who wants to do his own shopping is a much appreciated service. The home help needs to use tact and sensitivity; her service can be the one which enables an elderly person to feel that he is keeping his independence without having to ask family or neighbours for help, and therefore the job may include requests that are impractical or highly idiosyncratic but which must be responded to kindly. When home helps are able to do this, they promote a person's continuing independence in the community, and the organiser who backs up the home help service is a key person in community care.

Meals-on-Wheels

This streamlined version of the time-honoured act of taking a hot meal to an incapacitated neighbour is a vital part of any community's after-care services. Many severely handicapped elderly who live alone seem to be able to manage if they can get one meal a day. This service can be a temporary aid to someone who has lost kitchen skills after a period in hospital or following a stroke, but who is expected to regain strength or ability; or it can be established as a permanent household routine. The delivery of meals-on-wheels is often rushed and can occur in advance of lunchtime, and many people repudiate it on these grounds. The service is so helpful that continued refusal may indicate the presence of a more complex problem.

The elements of this provision are a kitchen, transport facilities and manpower. Voluntary organisations have often pioneered this service, offering coverage from 3 to 7 days a week. Overall availability of the service is more likely where a local authority or state body has opted for responsibility, supplementing existing facilities. Where such back-up does not exist and small community groups are losing their manpower for lack of resources (for instance fuel reimbursement money), then it is time for someone to intervene.

Both the home help service and the meals-on-wheels service form part of an unofficial safety check arrangement for the households at which they call. Limited access to communication facilities is one of the hardships in old age if physical mobility and financial independence are decreasing or already gone. A person who will take a message, whose visit can be counted on daily, is very important to the household.

Laundry Service for Incontinence

In addition to what the home helps can do in going out to a launderette or doing laundry at home, it can be very useful to have a specialised service for a household where there is incontinence. Local launderettes sometimes object to being used for this problem and severe domestic stress can result. This service is probably most helpful if it can be run on a collection and delivery basis; but fairly skilled persuasive tactics might be needed to induce a local organisation to offer the service, if the statutory agency is not already providing it.

Domiciliary Nursing and the General Practitioner

In a national health service, community medical care is carried out by a general practitioner, responsibility usually being determined roughly by geographical catchment. The GP and the public health nurse make up the basic team (primary health care team) in the community. In some instances there is also a social worker in the team. The general practitioner has a central role in caring for the elderly patients in his area. An enthusiastic doctor will not only be involved in the day-to-day care of acute problems but he will also be active in preventive aspects of health care in old age (Williams, 1979). As leader of the primary health care team in the community, he co-ordinates services for his elderly patients and he is also in a position to meet the challenging problem of unreported need (Chapter 2). In the absence of a GP system, something comparable needs to be available; perhaps a home care programme administered by the hospital, with contract arrangements for nursing services (Rossman and Burnside, 1975; Davidson and Marmor, 1980).

Fragmentation of service in community care for the elderly can be destructive. This age group is characterised by decreased resources of strength and money, and must let go by default the synthesis of health care that younger people can organise for themselves or obtain through employment group schemes. In the British system, where the nursing role is divided into two parts, the district nurse carries out nursing routines in the home and the health visitor, with a focus on health education, visits with information and advice, makes referrals, and is alert to issues of public health standards. The elderly in the community can benefit from both treatment and health advisory nursing services.

District Nurse

A domiciliary nurse who will carry out nursing procedures on a regular basis in the home is a vital part of the back-up services to a geriatric unit. At discharge, the geriatrician will hope to transfer care to the outside team which includes a nurse. It can be important in planning the strategic moment for someone's discharge to be able to hand over to the community nurse the continued treatment of leg ulcers, for instance, or the monitoring of a medication whose finer adjustment has not yet been stabilised. Because so many elderly people come in to hospital with multiple pathologies, it would be a pity if one continuing intransigent problem should prevent the discharge of someone whose treatment is otherwise complete, and for whom the right psychological moment for discharge has come.

The amount of labour and responsibility in nursing care which the hospital might pass on to the district nurse should be assessed in proportion to the resources available to the nurses in that community. In addition to nursing supplies and manpower, they will need the resource of the geriatric unit's quick response to requests for the re-admission of patients. Home nursing of the terminally ill is another service given by the district nurse in many areas. This may be the only way that a family can have its sick member at home with them.

Health Visitor

The health advisory aspect of community nursing is an important one for the progress of good health care for the elderly. The health visitor is a nurse with a post-registration qualification, the Health Visitor's Certificate. She is not engaged in practical nursing procedures but provides a health advisory service to families and individuals. The general public, in the main, subscribes to the view that nothing much can be done about the ills of old age. The health visitor can play an important role in changing these negative attitudes and she can also bring elderly people in the community with remediable conditions to the attention of the doctor. She may be asked to call by the GP, the social worker, the district nurse, a member of the public such as a neighbour or she may call on her own initiative. She can also mobilise other services for which a need is found, such as occupational therapy (OT) assessment, day care and so forth. This form of health care surveillance seems acceptable to a public accustomed to a national health service; whether it would fit in to other systems, socially and financially, is open to question.

A visitor with a specialist interest in the care of the elderly exists in some of the British health authority areas. There are many advantages in having a health visitor with this particular expertise. She can be an extremely helpful communication link between the unit and a patient's household. A pre-admission assessment of factors important to total patient care can be made available to the geriatrician if necessary (Chapter 2). Later, when discharge planning is under way, the health visitor can be invaluable in investigating and preparing domestic conditions before the patient returns. The independence someone achieves in hospital, in uncluttered corridors, away from kitchen hazards, and surrounded by personnel who will help him up from the floor, may be quite lost in the realities of his home. There mobility is restricted by furniture, toilets may be up or down steps or at the bottom of the garden, loose carpets interfere with the use of a walking aid, and no one calls for 8-hour stretches. Much of this side of patient treatment and preparation is covered of course by the occupational therapist, and it is a great help if there are community-based occupational therapists in addition to those who should form part of the geriatric hospital team. However, in many places the importance of the occupational therapist to geriatric care has not been sufficiently recognised and there is a shortage. It is often the health visitor who bridges the gap.

After a patient's discharge the health visitor can again help in communications. It is never certain whether a patient will be so delighted at getting home again that he will overcome monumental difficulties, or whether he will deteriorate, defeated by his handicap and his home's shortcomings and dismayed by the withdrawal of the hospital's supporting presence and personnel. The health visitor can assess this final and very important part of someone's treatment, and can alert the GP or the hospital if the situation is breaking down.

Domiciliary Physiotherapy

Continued supervised exercise is very important in some conditions found in the elderly. In a large or densely populated urban catchment area it might be worth examining the potential for obtaining the services of a domiciliary physiotherapist. Whilst a day hospital can meet the principal requirement for this service, some people may find the journey too difficult, or domestic arrangements may preclude their being able to use transport. Other potential users of such a service could well include homes for the elderly and nursing homes (Cronin, 1981).

Other Visitors

There is almost always good will in any community, which looks for ways of expression. To channel the impulse of people to be helpful, so that the help can benefit other community members without an atmosphere of patronage or charity, is an old challenge which needs to be faced if the elderly frail are to remain out of institutional care. Neighbourly goodwill cannot be demanded, but it is a necessary element in geriatric support services. If an organised scheme of support from the local health care authority can be seen to take responsibility, many informal services may be taken care of through neighbourliness. The vital job of calling in to see whether someone is all right will be performed as long as the caller can feel that the responsibility will not lie with him if things are found to be collapsing.

There are long-established organisations with a tradition of visiting whose administrative structure allows for the necessary support and advice to the visitors. Some social service departments in the UK have a formal arrangement for recruiting and supporting neighbourly volunteers. Camden's 'Good Neighbour' scheme pays an organiser to find, register, and then offer back-up support to the many people in the community who would like to take part informally. There is no task attached to the visit, and the health or daily maintenance of the person visited does not depend on the arrival of the Good Neighbour, who can therefore visit without undue burden of responsibility. The organiser is on the other end of the telephone if anything arises (Services for the Elderly, Camden, 1979).

A difficult assessment in the discharge planning for an elderly person living alone is calculating the necessary care or contact intervals (hourly, 3-hourly, 6-hourly) in the light of available visiting personnel. Not all contacts need be for task-performance, but after arrangements for home help, meals-on-wheels and domiciliary nursing, there may still be long hours unaccounted for, and particular circumstances may make the person concerned, or his community, feel that there is risk. This question is often subjective, but the involvement of visitors, even if they do not perform the heavy care tasks that a severely disabled person may require, can help greatly with the sharing of supervision.

Aids and Adaptations in the Home

There are a great many aids, some simple but very practical (like commodes), and some large and expensive (like bed hoists) which make it possible to consider home care for people with a wide range of difficulties. Some types of aid would be classed as useful devices for daily living activities, and the others consist of nursing aids and equipment. An excellent illustrated list can be found in *Caring for the Elderly Sick* (Chalmers, 1980).

It is also useful to have some way of helping patients to arrange for modifications to design problems in their housing. They may need minor adaptations carried out before they can return home: grab rails in the toilet and bath, additional rails on staircases; re-positioning of electric points to eliminate stooping; a small ramp to remove a one-step level change. The widening of a doorway for a wheelchair is a more serious undertaking. The setting up of a 'mini-hospital' in the home is controversial because of cost and the manpower needs involved (Evans, 1977), but our impression is that most community care programmes currently operating would include as necessities basic nursing aids, house safety aids, and activities of daily living (ADL) aids. Much of this falls to statutory provision in the UK; in other health care delivery systems it may be more complicated to locate these aids, many of which can make home a viable alternative to institutional care. A resource file, in the hospital, compiled with the help of the medical social workers and the occupational therapists, should be kept.

Specialised Clinic Services

Elderly people are quite likely to need ameliorative treatment to eyes,
ears, teeth and feet. The decline of these faithful servants is an insidious
affair. The sufferer is likely to have made involuntary adjustments to
the encroaching deficits until things have reached the point of accident,
isolation or malnutrition. This is an unconscious neglect. Foot care is a
fundamental element in mobility and independence which is often
given less attention than it warrants. Clinic services of optician, audio-
logist, dentist and chiropodist need to be available to the elderly section
of the population, regardless of financial means, if people are to make
the maximum use of their physical powers. A shortage of chiropodists
has been a handicap to many well-planned community care programmes.
In a national health scheme providing these specialised clinic services, it
is still necessary to examine carefully supply and demand. In other
health care frameworks, it will be very important to locate, and if
necessary develop, these specialties, and ensure their practical availability
to both inpatient and outpatient.

Health Centres

When planning services for the elderly it is always important to remember
that personal mobility and access to transport is often reduced. The
British plan of health centres locates centrally a group of services and
personnel. Any 'multi-purpose centre' is useful for a less mobile group
of customers. A health centre provides a base and telephone facilities for
members of the primary health care team. It also offers easy access to a
wide range of specialists: clinic nurse, health visitor, chiropodist,
ophthalmic, dental and aural specialists, a dietician and a physiotherapist.

Transport

Special transport for the physically handicapped is a great asset in a
community and one which is becoming more necessary as geriatric units
discharge people with increasingly greater degrees of handicap. In countries
where the health or social services have provided generously for this,
rising fuel costs are now beginning to weaken the service, but the
contribution which transport makes to someone's continued
independence at home is so important that communities must now

find ways of ensuring continuity.

Standard types of transport are those with ramps or tail-lifts to accommodate wheelchairs, and 'minibuses' which have a capacity for about 10 passengers and reasonably easy access via folding steps. Transport brings people to outpatient clinics, day hospitals, specialist services, lunch clubs, day centres and holiday outings, and takes the constriction out of the word 'housebound'. In the UK, the ambulance service usually makes vehicles available to day hospitals, while local authority clubs, centres and services use their own transport, under the Chronic Sick and Disabled Persons Act of 1970. If there is no hospital ambulance service, but rather private firms and health insurance contract systems, then it will be important to see whether the amenity is effectively available or whether it will need to be developed. If a geriatric unit with a day hospital can have its own ambulance or tail-lift van, many attendance problems can be eliminated. If people with severe degrees of handicap are to be enabled to remain at home with domiciliary supports, then specialised transport must be part of the system which sets out to make this idea practicable.

Ambulance crews should have special training to enable them to understand the needs of the older patient. This training should be broad based and include medical, social and psychological aspects as well as the use of modern devices which aid mobility. Departments of geriatric medicine should be willing to play an active part in developing such courses.

Day Centres

Some social centre facility to which transport is provided is a very useful resource. Any community will have its clubs and church groups and places where people get together for social contact. The more 'supportive' centres, which offer partial or complete day care, exist to provide the facilities of a club plus support during the day for those in difficult circumstances at home (Morley, 1979).

A day centre can offer a selection of active and passive occupations, and provide a lunch. It has a fairly high level of attendant staff to assist handicapped members in the activities of daily living. It may offer chiropody, washing machine and dryer facilities, hairdressing, baths, and a public telephone. Depending on the nature of its community, it can also link up with local adult education amenities and offer courses in both academic subjects and arts and crafts. A day centre makes an important contribution to the provision of home care. A supervised bath for example at the day centre may be more practical than a struggle for a home health aide in a house with unsuitable bath facilities.

Adequate day care resources make home life for the very dependent elderly much easier; the family or the community caring personnel can undertake a heavier commitment if there is a possibility of weekly relief. A geriatric day hospital will need to be able to find social substitutes for the contacts and friendships its patients will have made during their treatment. Many elderly people will have their first experience of the social club atmosphere when attending a day hospital and will find it a lifeline that cannot be relinquished when medical treatment is at an end. Under these circumstances the possibility of transferring a person from day hospital attendance to day centre attendance in the community can be very valuable.

Lunch Clubs

A less complicated amenity for providing food and company is the lunch club. Contemporary employment patterns have accustomed many of us to an arrangement where we join friends or colleagues for convenience and pleasure whilst eating. The frail elderly may have lost the contacts which would enable them to continue the natural conjunction of food and society, and the tea and toast syndrome, resulting in severe nutritional deficiencies, is an understandable response to a task that is both impractical and tedious.

The elderly living alone are particularly vulnerable if their solitude is the result of loss. Like the day centre, the lunch club contains the element of social support, and premises should be suitable for the handicaps of age. As a resource, it is more easily organised, needing less capital outlay, personnel and time. It can develop out of existing club systems that cater for other age groups. It can link up with day centres (whose kitchens can be used) and with a meals-on-wheels service (whose distribution system can bring prepared food to a central point).

Residential Care

The frail elderly who are fortunate in living in well-balanced communities having neighbourliness, convenient shops, good public transport, housing for all income levels, and stability, will more easily manage to remain supported in their homes. An area that is deficient in some or all of these qualities may find itself needing purpose-built housing which, being planned essentially for the convenience of the helpers, may be quite uncongenial to the residents for whom it is ostensibly designed.

The elderly (the least mobile of us) are likely to be left in poor housing, as younger people move to something more convenient. An older generation accepts from habit and custom conditions that make life awkward: fifth-floor walk-ups, outside toilets, narrow ill-lit passages, or uneven stone-flagged floors. For a small percentage of the patients in a geriatric unit, a return home to the living arrangements from which they came, even with support services and adaptation or rehousing, and family care, will not be feasible. They will need social care and attention. There comes a point in the assessment of potential for continuing to live at home, when the care needed exceeds what the family or community can give. In the UK, residential or long-stay accommodation is the solution usually put forward at this stage.

A residential home undertakes to provide meals, housekeeping, laundry, etc., and a responsible person on duty at all times. Supervision can be provided at hazard points: in the bath, on stairs; and help is available for dressing and toileting if necessary. A considerable degree of frailty is usually tolerated, but staffing patterns do not generally include nurses. This resource, a statutory obligation on local authority social service departments, is augmented by private and voluntary homes and seems to meet a demand for care facilities for people who do not require active medical or nursing care, but simply supervised living conditions and, if necessary, help with ADL.

In communities which undertake to provide a good network of community care services, a combination of factors has altered the nature of residential care, or the 'old folks' home'. In the first place there are now more frail old people. Increased domiciliary manpower is available to people wishing to remain at home, so that when someone decides that he cannot manage at home, he probably requires a fair amount of supervision, or even nursing. However, residential homes have been planned to emphasise the element 'home', and do not offer, in equipment or staffing, facilities for heavy nursing. The voluntary homes find that this qualitative change in their potential residents poses a financial problem (NCCOP/Age Concern, 1977). State-supported institutions, less flexible in adapting to change though sometimes more shock-absorbent financially, having changed from the 500-bed institutional pattern to the small home of 40-60 beds, also find it troublesome that people applying for residential facilities often need quite extensive care. It is important to be aware of the original purposes of local long-stay resources, as well as to know their present structural and staffing arrangements.

The emphasis, in Britain, is on getting a person out of the hospital setting and back into the community, and the residential homes are seen as part of the community, thus making an important distinction between two life-styles. They were designed to provide homes for people, not treatment for patients. In contrast, the American post-hospital long-term care resource seems to be the nursing home. Here the hospital medical model is consciously followed and community life-style appears to be relinquished in favour of an environment of protection from health relapse or illness.

Ironically, the regime in many British residential homes makes residents increasingly dependent and eventually unwilling to do things for themselves (Gibberd, 1977). The degree of care that has to be offered to the less able residents encourages the more able to become dependent and to expect the same degree of support. In one area the officers in charge of local authority homes suggested that some of their residents would have been better placed in sheltered accommodation but that after a period in the home they no longer had the inclination to cope for themselves (DHSS, 1979). A careful medical and social assessment to prevent inappropriate placement is therefore essential before people take up permanent residence in institutional accommodation. It is also important to assess the institution, because every establishment develops its own personality, and its physical and social qualities may be unsuited to a prospective resident who would settle perfectly well into a different but equally protective setting elsewhere.

Brocklehurst *et al.* (1978) discovered a significant number of people suffering from remediable illness when they assessed the residents of a number of homes. They concluded that all people seeking institutional care should be examined carefully to exclude treatable pathology as a reason for their inability to cope at home.

Sheltered Housing

An acceptable alternative to full residential care for the more able is the 'sheltered housing' unit, which exists in many forms and has proved a very effective preserver of home continuity and independence for elderly people. Self-contained living units are grouped together and usually have a resident warden or supervisor. The function of the latter is to be on the alert in case any household is in difficulties, and to supervise more or less closely, depending upon local wishes and so forth, the welfare of each household.

A daily check call may be made by the warden; or alternatively a call-button system operated by the householder may be preferred. People are responsible for their own housekeeping (and this includes the services of home helps and meals-on-wheels in areas where such exist). The degree of supervisory function in the role of the warden can be varied as need arises. Call buttons, warning lights, two-way intercoms, and many informal arrangements are used to care for less active elderly people, whilst informal arrangements between tenants can develop as an effective self-help system. The use of warden communication systems can also help in enabling frail elderly people to remain in their own homes.

The present level of provision of sheltered housing is totally inadequate in most areas (Chapter 2). Because of this many old people have no option but to enter residential accommodation when disability makes it impossible for them to continue living in housing which has become inadequate for their needs. Progress in Britain in this field has been hampered by administrative difficulties because sheltered housing is provided by the Department of the Environment and local authority housing departments, and not by the DHSS and social services departments.

It becomes apparent, after a geriatric unit has been operating for some years, that it is helpful to have aftercare institutions of three different types: long-stay nursing facilities, residential homes and sheltered housing. The shortage of any one of these seems to result in the abuse of the others, to the grave detriment of the quality of life for people using the facility.

The Geriatric Unit and the Community

A geriatric unit should be as close as possible to its community, and the partnership between it and those that care for the frail elderly at home should be based on good understanding. Families and hardworking community service personnel will put up with very taxing and sometimes unbelievable burdens of care if stress, leading to desperation, can be avoided. In fact, help is needed well before crisis point, because people who are looking after frail and often difficult elderly people at home will probably exhaust their emotional and even physical resources before something happens to precipitate hospital admission. The caring household may then be unable to resume so destructive a burden, and the hospital patient becomes homeless. There are two main ways in which a geriatric unit can be of service in these situations.

Short-period admissions of the patient whose home care involves heavy nursing can give the caring agent a chance to rest, to attend to personal business, or to have a holiday, and will probably in the long run release more beds for active treatment use (Chapter 3). Readmission for intensive rehabilitation, to restore necessary mobility or to adjust sensitive medications, should be readily available to patients. It is very important for families and domiciliary visiting personnel to know that the hospital will hear and respond to a cry for help. The onus is on the hospital to build up the trust which will allow the community to care for severely handicapped and frail elderly in their homes. The intensive discharge policy implicit in geriatric rehabilitation has contributed to the altered balance of care in the community, and the geriatric unit should be sensitive to this (Baker and Hargreaves, 1980).

The second way in which a geriatric unit can help indirectly in home care is in promoting as much as possible good communications between itself and those working in the community. It is important to observe the basic courtesy of adequate notice of discharges where community help will be enlisted. There are also many details of the daily living routines of a patient that are taken for granted in the ward setting which will not be the same in home circumstances. Most of us behave one way in an institution, and quite differently on our own territory. The occupational therapist is always alert to this fact, but all hospital staff need to develop awareness of the implications for their own discipline. A good way to resolve what can be enormously complex differences of opinion between hospital, patient, and outside caring agent, is to arrange case conferences, where all the protagonists can meet together and agree, or agree to disagree. (This possibility must be recognised and allowed.) A conference can bring together the hospital team, the district nurse, the home help organiser, representatives of voluntary agencies whose personnel may be giving supportive time and care to a patient, and last, but not least, the person whose discharge is being arranged.

A geriatric service has an educational function implicit in its belief that good acute medicine is as much the right of the very old as of any other age category. This is still a new idea. The hospital can also contribute more directly to in-service training programmes for many of the service professions whose work involves contact with the elderly. Many of the 'unskilled' levels of staff in all places where the elderly are served are deprived of opportunities to learn about and understand the special problems of old age. Day hospital premises are ideal early evening meeting places; when the patients have been taken home at the end of the day, a useful community resource becomes available. There are many other ways in which both hospital and community can serve as resources for one another and each will benefit from co-operative ventures of this nature.

References

Age Concern (1980). *Age Concern at Work*. Age Concern, London

Baker, M.R. and Hargreaves, E. (1980). 'Health and Social Service Planning'. *Public Health*, 94, 5, 306

Brocklehurst, J.C., Carty, M.H., Leeming, J.T. and Robinson, J.M. (1978). 'Medical Screening of old people accepted for residential care'. *Lancet*, 2, 141

Chalmers, G.L. (1980). *Caring for the Elderly Sick*. Pitman, London

Cronin, C. (1981). 'Domiciliary Physiotherapy: a Complementary Service'. *Geriatric Medicine*, 11, 79

Davidson, S.M. and Marmor, T.R. (1980). *The Cost of Living Longer*. Lexington Press, Massachusetts

Department of Health and Social Security (1979). *Residential Care for the Elderly in London*. DHSS, London

Evans, J.G. (1977). 'Current Issues in the United Kingdom', in *Care of the Elderly*, A.N. Exton-Smith and J.G. Evans (eds.). Academic Press, London, and Grune and Stratton, New York

Gibberd, K. (1977). *Home For Life. What Alternatives?* Age Concern, London

Lipman, V. (1959). *A Century of Social Service 1858-1959*. Routledge and Kegan Paul, London

Morley, D. (1979). *Day Care*. Age Concern, London

National Corporation for the Care of Old People and Age Concern (1977). *Extra Care?* Age Concern, London

Rossman, I. and Burnside, I.M. (1975). 'The United States of America', in *Geriatric Care in Advanced Societies*, J.C. Brocklehurst (ed.). M.T.P., Lancaster; University Park Press, Baltimore

Services for the Elderly in Camden (1979). Annual publication, Department of Social Services, Camden, London

Williams, I. (1979). *The Care of the Elderly in the Community*. Croom Helm, London

10 DEVELOPING A PSYCHOGERIATRIC SERVICE

D. Jolley, P. Smith, L. Billington, D. Ainsworth and D. Ring

Hospitals

The hospitals that serve most English towns and cities had their origins in previous centuries. They reflect in durable brick and mortar and in almost equally durable professional organisation, the requirements of a population very different from that which lives in England today. Centrally placed and carrying high kudos is the former 'voluntary' or 'acute' hospital v .h an established expectation that patients are accepted with acute illnesses from which they will die or recover in response to treatment. Elsewhere, often in a poorer part of the town, the chronic sickness hospital has performed loyal service to those unfortunates struck down by tuberculosis or other similarly debilitating illness. Further off again, maybe in the local countryside or a distant moor, the County Asylum is whispered of with awe and known to children as a place of nightmares and fascinating chastisement.

The Population

In previous centuries the population was smaller and suffered illnesses that often led to death in infancy or relative youth. As recently as 1900 only 5 per cent of the population was aged 65 years or older. Young people usually have the decency to fall ill with one illness at a time, thus it was not inappropriate that one institution dealt with pneumonia, dysentry, heart failure and the like, another institution catered for tuberculosis and a third provided for the mentally disordered suffering from schizophrenia, general paralysis of the insane and manic depressive psychosis.

The success of public health measures associated with industrially produced wealth has changed all this (McKeown, 1976). People are now very heavily concentrated into urban areas; thus the countryside is in many instances no more populous than in previous centuries but towns are very much bigger. The increase in population is almost entirely attributable to greater life expectancy among infants and young people. The infections that afflicted these age groups and which took them to hospitals and the grave have become rare as a result of better sanitation, better ventilation and improved resistance in a better fed population. Today most babies will be expected to live into the seventh decade and beyond. The introduction of effective chemotherapy over the past 40 years has meant that bacterial infections can usually be treated quickly and effectively without recourse to hospitalisation. In those severe cases where hospital admission is still necessary, most will return home in a matter of days.

Old Age

Old age brings with it an expectation of disability produced by an accumulation of pathologies, some long standing, others arising for the first time in the senium, some physical, others emotional or mental. Disabilities are thrown cruelly into perspective by the social character-istics that mark out old age as a time of relative poverty during which an individual is more likely to be living alone or with one other equally old and potentially disabled person than in a larger family (Hunt, 1978).

The additive effects of physical, mental and social difficulties lead some old people to require help from others if they are to survive. When this need escalates beyond that which can be mobilised at home, the hospital services with their tripartite historical structure are ill con-stituted to provide an appropriate response.

Current practice often uses the terms 'old' or 'elderly' as equivalent to 'retirement' age or 65 years. This device of defining 'old age' by chronological arbitration is convenient for administrative purposes but broadens the concept away from longer-established usage which includes the notion of functional decline and enfeeblement. Thus statistical descriptions of 'old age' defined chronologically are less poignant than they might be. For whilst 95 per cent of people over 65 years live in private households, the proportion falls rapidly within the eighth and ninth decades and within each decade is much smaller for disabled people (Clarke *et al.*, 1979). Thus chronic sickness hospitals have been largely taken over by the elderly. Half of all mental hospital beds are occupied by old people and even within 'acute' or 'general' hospitals up to half the beds are used for the elderly. Similarly within welfare establishments organised under Part III of the National Assistance Act there are accumulations of increasingly old and disabled residents (Wilkin *et al.*, 1978).

Psychiatry and Geriatric Medicine

Reviewing the functions of mental illness and chronic sickness hospitals, McKeown *et al.* (1961) pointed out that many of their elderly patients shared characteristics of physical and mental frailty. Since that time chronic sickness hospitals have been actively developed to form the basis of geriatric services, a process described elsewhere within this book. Psychiatric services have been changing, too, for while independent mental hospitals were being built and expanded up to the Second World War, this pattern has since been reversed and every mental hospital boasted a graph of declining residence rates and looked forward to its eventual extinction. Two major movements have contributed to this contraction of the mental hospitals (Jolley, 1976a). The first has been the creation of psychiatric units in general hospitals, stressing the affinity of psychiatry with the rest of medicine and assuming the medical model of illness and curability for many of its afflictions. The second has been the philosophy of 'community care', suggesting that removal from the normal world is antitherapeutic and maintenance within the community is always preferable and usually possible. The swing towards 'psychological medicine' as practised in general hospital units has, perhaps perversely, directed the interests of many psychiatrists away from the elderly. For the dementing illnesses which are common only among the elderly do not conform to the curability model that has been applied to mood disorders and other psychoses. In addition the multidimensional problems presented by old people sometimes require hospital care including some long-term care that runs counter to the self-imposed need of psychiatry to cope with fewer beds than in the past. The contrast between the unfashionable toil and care required by the elderly and the more immediate rewards obtained among some younger psychiatric patients has led to the view that 'they do not require the skills of a [modern] psychiatrist'.

Many of the old people accumulating in mental hospitals are residents of long-stay wards and as such unlikely to be seen frequently by a doctor, particularly a consultant. In many instances the training and personal skills of nursing staff responsible for their care are only tangentially related to the needs of the patients. Thus within the alternative society of the mental hospital, the elderly are particularly vulnerable to hazards which have given rise to a series of scandals followed by official inquiries.

Yet the significance of old age for the practice of psychiatry in the latter half of the twentieth century has been predictable and predicted

(Lewis, 1946). Even within the late forties and fifties individual psychiatrists had declared a real interest in the elderly and had grappled with their requirements. Thus Post began a series of clinical studies that have spanned 30 years (Post, 1978). Roth's meticulous analysis of old people admitted to mental hospitals was extended in association with Kay and others in Newcastle. Their studies provided a firm foundation for the epidemiology of mental disorders in old age and a more comprehensive understanding of the use of services by their patients (Roth, 1955; Kay *et al.*, 1964).

Psychogeriatric Services

Meanwhile MacMillan had tuned the Nottingham psychiatric service based at Mapperley Hospital to be particularly responsive to the needs of the elderly and to work closely with others (notably the social services) who were similarly interested in this group (MacMillan, 1960). His initiative in England was mirrored in Scotland by Robinson's Crichton Royal service (Robinson, 1962). Sainsbury's classical evaluation of the 'community orientated' psychiatric service in Chichester noted the success of this approach in making contact with the elderly and enabling them to manage or be managed without recourse to mental hospital (Sainsbury *et al.*, 1965).

These were trail blazing, often isolated, ventures. The relationship between the newly emerging specialty of geriatric medicine and the changling new psychiatry was not clear and in some areas was frankly hostile. Kidd's appraisal of practice in Belfast suggested that whilst the majority of new admissions to the two specialties were correctly placed, some were seriously misplaced and many patients had mixed problems with both physical and mental components (Kidd, 1962). Investigation of admissions elsewhere have confirmed that many patients have both physical and mental problems, though the incidence of serious misplacement is generally agreed to be minimal. This situation moved the Department of Health to promote the development of psychogeriatric units to facilitate collaboration between psychiatrists, geriatricians and social service workers (DHSS, 1970). In addition the role of psychiatric services in providing for the elderly was outlined in a separate document whose main purpose appears to have been to perpetuate the *status quo* as reflected by superficial data that included no estimate of quality of service (Jolley, 1977). Thankfully this does not appear to have done a great deal of harm, though it is doubtful if it has achieved much good and the time is surely ripe for a redesigned statement of policy, enlightened by developments during the seventies.

Among those drawn to create psychogeriatric services, several have been gifted evangelists and publicists. Tony Whitehead, recently pictured accompanying a hover mower from London to Brighton, has a practised gift for catching the public eye; Brice Pitt's easily read book has introduced many to the essential issues (Pitt, 1974); and the charm and intellect of Tom Arie added fascination to the messages made plain by Klaus Bergman, Gordon Langley, Gary Blessed and others. Those early into the field made provision for mutual support by creating a special-interest group within the Royal College of Psychiatrists. Starting in 1974 with a few members and meeting regularly every quarter, this group has succoured newcomers who have been able to share their trials and frustrations and benefit from the experience of others. Many members have been encouraged to join the British Geriatrics Society and the lively interaction between the BGS and this group has been very fruitful. In addition the group addressed itself to particular topics and produced a series of policy documents as well as spawning a number of conferences and research initiatives. By 1979 the membership had reached such numbers that the group was granted Section status within the Royal College of Psychiatrists, and is expected to continue to develop in influence and potential. Thus from the sporadic developments of the fifties and sixties, the seventies have produced a situation where more than a hundred consultant psychiatrists are said to view the elderly as their main interest and responsibility (Wattis *et al.*, 1980).

Styles of Psychogeriatric Service

A variety of styles has always been identifiable within the psychogeriatric movement (Jolley and Arie, 1978). All seek to act as a focus to facilitate the psychiatric contribution to care of the elderly within the spectrum of caring available within the locality. The detailed development and function of individual services depends on local circumstances, including the historical balance of provision, the prevailing political scene and the presence of motivated, interested professionals.

Probably the commonest pattern is that which starts from a large mental hospital wherein a number of wards occupied by old people become the springboard for a community-orientated service that establishes links with local geriatric units and social services. Frequently the number of beds in use is reduced so that overcrowding is avoided and ward milieu is improved and sometimes day care activities are linked to the invigorated wards. It is unusual for all old people in a mental hospital to come within the psychogeriatric service, for many have graduated into old age as chronic psychotics and remain with their established firms. The new approach is directed towards the particular needs of people falling ill within old age, though there is little doubt that many 'graduates' share the physical frailties of this group and do benefit when account is taken of this. A few psychogeriatricians are convinced that all elderly people in psychiatric care should be accommodated within the psychogeriatric service and in the future this lobby may well hold sway, for fewer people will grow old in mental hospitals and more will present within the community scarred by illnesses that had their roots earlier in life. Mental hospitals were not built with old people in mind. Most now serve enormous catchment areas and catchment populations and are situated many miles from their potential clientele and families. Buildings are old, large, poorly lit and difficult to heat. Toilets and bathing areas are only suitable for physically able tenants. Recruitment into psychogeriatric nursing has been alarmingly poor in recent years and the training that many receive emphasises the interest and reward obtained from nursing 'acute' patients. Involvement of nurse therapists in the treatment of neurotic problems and the aggrandisement of psychotherapeutic techniques in general may seem to direct the nurse away from the elderly. In fact minor modifications of these very skills make for entirely appropriate techniques in psychogeriatric practice. Yet it remains (understandably) difficult to recruit suitable nurses and maintain their morale on long-stay wards of isolated mental hospitals. What has been said of nurses is more emphatically true of occupational therapists and physiotherapists. It is not unusual for hundreds of disabled old people to be housed in a mental hospital where no occupational therapy time is given to the elderly and where physiotherapists are unknown.

In some areas psychogeriatric services have developed from a geriatric hospital base. They may have the advantage of close association with a driving geriatric service yet the psychiatric team may feel isolated and misunderstood away from their co-professionals. Again the buildings may be ill equipped, particularly in providing for the more vigorous ambulant patient. Nurse training, though likely to include a thorough appreciation of physical needs and appropriate skills, may lack something in understanding emotional needs and the techniques for coping with and modifying sustained distressed or distressing behaviour.

Relatively few services have developed from a general hospital base with a full range of medical specialties including general psychiatry and geriatric medicine. Yet this is probably an ideal situation and one we have been fortunate to explore in South Manchester.

Development of the Psychogeriatric Service in South Manchester

Origins

South Manchester Health District spans the River Mersey and is the largest of three districts which have constituted Manchester Area Health Authority (Teaching) since the reorganisation of the Health Service in 1974 (Figure 10.1). The resident population of roughly 200,000 includes 28,000 aged 65 years and older. Social service provision is through Manchester City Corporation and administered through three area teams (areas 4, 5 and 6 of Manchester SS). Withington Hospital is the largest general hospital in the district and is a major teaching hospital: the University Hospital of South Manchester. It includes a Department of Psychiatry which has served the resident population as well as providing undergraduate and postgraduate teaching since 1971. The Department of Geriatric Medicine has been an established part of the hospital for many years and since 1970 has included a professorial unit. There is another large general hospital, Wythenshaw Hospital, within the district and this has a smaller geriatric unit.

Prior to the opening of the psychiatric unit at Withington, psychiatric services to the district had been provided by Prestwich Hospital and/or Springfield Hospital – mental hospitals to the north of the city. The unit provides 160 beds and an 80-place day hospital together with out-patient facilities to serve the local population. It also accepts some patients from further afield in keeping with its teaching hospital function. Although the unit determined to provide a 'comprehensive' response to the community's needs, it followed the precedent set by other units in the North West in expecting to avoid responsibility for the long-term care of people suffering from dementia. The department of geriatric medicine was serving a much larger catchment population (roughly 52,000 elderly) and, like many other geriatric services, was used to dealing with a number of patients suffering from dementia. It is probably true to say that most old people who needed hospital care whether because of physical or mental frailty would be referred to a geriatrician unless they were obviously depressed or paranoid and had no evidence of dementia. Very few elderly people from South Manchester were admitted to Prestwich or Springfield hospitals after 1970, only the most disturbed cases being referred on by the geriatricians. In

Figure 10.1: The Manchester Health District

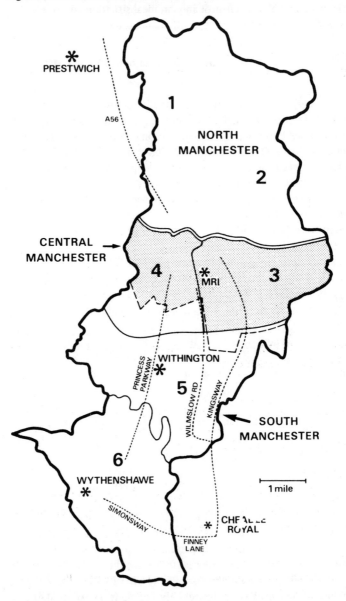

keeping with this situation the geriatric department had acquired a
block of 42 beds at a small private mental hospital (Cheadle Royal)

for the management of long-stay dementing women.

Despite good will on all sides these arrangements were felt to be imperfect and it became a recurring embarrassment that general practitioners found difficulty in placing elderly patients when mental disorder contributed to their being at risk or in distress in the community. Thus it was decided to establish a psychogeriatric service.

The Facilities

The following facilities were provided:

Withington Hospital Department of Psychiatry

10 beds (2 beds each from the existing 5 firms, distributed between 4 different wards. All but 2 of these beds were occupied by patients who were believed to be dementing and had been in hospital for 6 months or more);
10 day places;
Outpatient facilities;
Use of a small office.

Department of Geriatric Medicine

An aged, dilapidated pavilion which had housed 77 long-stay patients had been emptied by opening extra wards at Withington and Wythenshawe hospitals. Plans had been drawn up to upgrade this building to accommodate 44 inpatients.

Cheadle Royal Hospital

42 beds (these were occupied by 42 established patients, all women suffering from dementia. The annual patient flow since 1972 had stabilised at 12 deaths, 12 admissions.)

The Beginnings

Starting in November 1975 there was no designated personnel other than the consultant. The role envisaged for the service, based on a year's study of services throughout the country (Jolley, 1976b) was:

To respond to the needs of patients over the age of 65 years referred from the catchment population of the Department of Psychiatry with mental disorders of any sort unless they were specifically referred to another psychiatrist who was willing to accept them. Certainly all patients suffering from dementia would be accepted and there should be no lower age limit to their referral.

Thus it was hoped to cater for all dements and all elderly people suffering from mental disorders, unless a specific wish had been confirmed that another consultant would take them on. Referrals were accepted from the first day in November; no special publicity was arranged. An essential and sustained philosophy was that the best service that could be offered within the constraints of existing facilities was the only meaningful aim possible. Within these constraints the concept of a waiting list constituted no service at all and was therefore not a mode of action to be accepted. It was important to monitor the service given to allow analysis of the management offered as some of it would inevitably be judged less than ideal by those providing it.

Secretarial Support. This was the first achievement facilitated by the administration. A competent interested secretary became and remains a central cog in the developing machinery of service. All referrals are channelled through her by phone, letter or word of mouth. We designed a referral card to standardise the request for information of social as well as clinical circumstances. These cards provide a manageable source of information within the office that can be supplemented by recourse to bulkier notes stored in the records department when appropriate. In addition the card information is easily coded for storage by computer which means analysis of activity is quite straightforward.

Social Work Support. No formal arrangements regarding social work support had been made before the consultant began to work. Fortunately the senior social worker appointed to the department of geriatric medicine during the same month had previous experience and a great interest in mentally ill old people. She negotiated a role that allowed her to spend time with the psychogeriatric service as well as fulfil her commitments to the geriatric unit. In practice she was doing at least two fulltime jobs at the same time.

Psychiatric Nurse Working in the Community. Again no formal arrangements had been agreed but the hospital-based community psychiatric nurses were interested in helping the new service and one nurse in particular began to take on large numbers of patients.

We had then the essentials for a team: doctor, social worker, psychiatric nurse in the community and secretary (with records system). There were three areas of work to be undertaken:

1. To deal as well as possible with new referrals, recognising the limits set by our meagre resources.
2. To assess and, if necessary and possible, improve the use of the resources already available to us as well as encourage the provision of others.
3. To explore the existing areas of support available to our potential patients with a view to identifying ways in which we could work with them.

Our knowledge of the geriatric unit (and their knowledge of us) was already extensive as the consultant had worked with them during the previous year and the social worker continued her role within that unit. In addition attendance at the established liaison meeting in the geriatric unit broadened our contact with area social workers, district nurse liaison officers, health visitors, and others.

A relationship with the social services was pursued by setting aside every Tuesday afternoon to visit and discuss matters with area teams. This led us to close contact with social workers and the staff of residential homes. It was clear that social services were managing a tremendous number of mentally ill old people both by domiciliary support and within their residential homes. These latter were a source of never ending inspiration to us. We learned a good deal of very good practice from the officers in charge and other staff. Their skills in managing disabled old people as well as coping with the complexities of managing small institutions and raising funds and interest in the locality were beyond all reasonable expectation. We were able to add our interest and developing expertise to this established pool of caring. There were numerous and increasing interactions with our colleagues and gradually an acceptable mutual understanding and respect emerged. This could never be achieved by chairbound discussions.

Bed Allocation. The dispersal of our beds at Withington through four different wards with a fraction share of four sets of junior doctors was a major disadvantage. There was no doubting the reason behind this fragmentation. It was not that every ward was keen to have us, rather that none wanted us with the image of incurability, physical dependence, non-communication and incontinence that characterised our inheritance. Yet to change this image through an effort spread over four wards, on each of which we represented but one-sixteenth of the bed allocation, was a difficult prospect. By a combination of careful attention to the patients, minimal improvements in their condition and our own vigorously

exposed interest and commitment to them some progress was made.
After a number of meetings six patients were brought together on one
ward and four on another. This with the prospect of a few 'loaned' beds
kept us 'afloat' for two years. During this time the Withington psychiatric unit, with its open-plan wards, divan beds, and nurses dressed in
civilian clothes, represented our only general hospital beds. As such it
served to provide assessment and treatment of confused, sometimes
incontinent, as well as functionally ill old people. Space to accept
admissions was engineered by transfer of female patients to Cheadle
Royal as vacancies were created by deaths in the post-Christmas period
of 1976. Perhaps our greatest strength lay in the unit at Cheadle Royal.
For though the ward was too big with 42 very disabled patients and had
no pretentions to achieve a 'turnover', the nursing and occupational
therapy staff had created a model regime. All the principles that one
might preach about the optimal management of dementing people were
there provided for daily demonstration.

Referrals

During the first 14 months (November 1975-December 1976) we
received roughly 500 new referrals. Half were at home and were visited
there at the request of the general practitioner, the remainder were
visited on wards at Withington and other hospitals at the request of
physicians, surgeons, geriatricians, etc. In most instances assessment
led to advice and sometimes suggestions regarding medication. Only 70
admissions were possible within this first year and all of these were to
the 10 beds at Withington. Day hospital attendances were limited to 5 each
day, partly out of consideration for transport, but also to avoid straining
the nurses beyond the possibilities of their inappropriate resources. The
Psychiatric Day Hospital at Withington was ill suited to manage confused
people, especially if they need help at toilet.

There is no doubt that the patients, their relatives, our co-professionals and we ourselves were under considerable pressure. However the Area
Medical Officer found that the number of complaints from general
practitioners fell remarkably. Those patients who needed assessment
and treatment for non-organic mental disorders got it, through work
with them at home, supplemented by outpatient attendance and
occasionally admission. Those patients who needed assessment and
treatment for obviously acute organic psychosyndromes got it, often
with help from a geriatrician. The chronic progressive dementing
syndromes were assessed at home and further investigation was arranged
through the outpatient clinic. Extra support offered had to be carefully

titrated. In every instance the rule had to be that 'the least extra that allows acceptable coping represents the best use of resources'. Thus regular visits to a tiring husband might be sufficient. If he needed time to himself, day hospital attendance or daytime attendance at a residential home was arranged and often surprised us by stimulating the dementing partner to greater self interest. People living alone and failing to cope because of dementia needed careful consideration. Sometimes adding to the support from home help or meals-on-wheels and neighbourhood warden was enough. A few lone dementing women remain able to manage with this sort of help for years. More require to move into a residential home, but only rarely did this need to be done via hospital.

By the end of 1976 the pattern of work had become established and 140 patients were carried into the New Year, living at home but receiving support, treatment and monitoring through our 'continuing care' domiciliary activities. The second full year of the service, 1977, was one of consolidation and preparation. Thus the character of referrals remained similar, though with the inheritance from 1976 more patients were handled than in the previous year. Within our existing resources it became possible to use vacancies that arose at Cheadle Royal more actively. Thus for the first time this unit began to discharge patients. At the same time men were allowed into what became a mixed sex ward.

The potential of an outpatient clinic for assessment of patients jointly with a geriatrician had become apparent and a lengthy series of negotiations were made to obtain facilities for this within the main out-patient block at Withington. In addition the upgrading of the ward block vacated by the geriatric unit was proceeding and careful attention to the details of this were necessary to ensure the best outcome. The plans made provision for a physiotherapy area and a kitchen for occupational therapy activities. The need for a day hospital for patients suffering from dementia was recognised but no definite scheme had been accepted into the planning programme. We decided to reduce the number of beds available on the ground floor to provide day space which would be used by daytime attenders as well as residents until such time as a definitive day hospital could be provided. This decision has proved to be very important as this makeshift 'day hospital' is central to the effective use of the unit.

A senior registrar from the pool of trainees in psychiatry had been attached to us. We were able to offer him a lively training experience and he strengthened our clinical team. Now a nursing officer joined us and together with an administrative assistant, added drive and know-how to the demanding task of commissioning the upgraded building and recruiting staff to work in it. Our work in the community had increased and a second community psychiatric nurse began to work with us. Our hard-pressed social worker achieved further funding for colleagues to share her workload.

When we came to recruit nursing staff for the upgraded unit there was insufficient money to open both floors. Thus we had to choose between an assessment ward or a continuing-care ward linked to the makeshift day hospital. There seemed little sense in opening an assessment ward with less than reasonable continuing-care facilities, so the decision was made. Suitable senior nursing staff were sought and it is worth reporting that two of the three sisters appointed were returning to hospital work after a period in local authority residential homes. We were fortunate in appointing an occupational therapist who has gathered round her a team of aides and trainees. Similarly the hospital physiotherapists have given us stimulating service from the beginning.

The team now had the additional potential of 20 continuing-care beds linked to 10 day attendances. Thirteen of these beds were given over to established long-stay demented patients from the Withington psychiatric unit and those few patients who had been admitted to Prestwich Hospital from South Manchester since 1970. This was done to avoid any massive escalation in expectations from this long-stay facility. The changes allowed 7 beds to be used for assessment and treatment of organic psychosyndromes and from that time onwards no 'confused' patients have been managed in the psychiatric unit at Withington. The 10 beds we retain in the psychiatric unit have been used for elderly people with non-organic psychosyndromes. It quickly became apparent that this group was welcome on a ward shared with the patients of a general psychiatrist.

Our established patient load of 300 was carried with lighter heart into 1978. We received a further 360 new referrals into the service during that year, having access to more appropriate inpatient and day patient accommodation as well as the benefits of assessment in an outpatient clinic run jointly with the Department of Geriatric Medicine (Jolley *et al.*, 1980).

Yet the main purpose of the service was to maintain close interaction with social services, geriatric medicine and primary health care services in order to support a large number of people at home or in other non-hospital accommodation. This philosophy has continued through 1979 when extra funds allowed the opening of the inpatient assessment ward. It functions well in providing intensive investigation, assessment and treatment, facilitated by regular ward rounds with a physician in geriatric medicine. We now have the equivalent of one full-time social worker as part of our team who deals with clients from each of the local authority areas. We are moving towards linking each social worker with a community psychiatric nurse. These 'duos' have a thorough knowledge of local facilities, are well known to other professionals in the area and are able to link the work of the area with us in a 'community-round' every week.

Further Developments

It is hoped to provide a definitive day hospital linked to the psycho-geriatric unit at Withington Hospital. A purpose-built unit with inpatient and day patient facilities is envisaged for Wythenshawe Hospital so that the populations on either side of the Mersey can be served more appropriately. This would allow our withdrawal from Cheadle Royal Hospital.

In addition our first senior registrar, now a consultant in North Manchester, has been developing a service there based on available mental hospital beds. A productive series of negotiations initiated by the Health Care Planning Team for Mental Illness in Central Manchester has created the probability that a service will begin there in the near future. This will be based in a health centre until such time (planned 1983) as facilities are built at Manchester Royal Infirmary.

Teaching. We have been fortunate in having the opportunity to teach a wide range of professionals. This is an opportunity to share our enthusiasm and awakening expertise with others who have the potential to do a great deal for old people. Medical students and postgraduate psychiatrists in training have been involved with us from the beginning. General practitioners and physicians in geriatric medicine are involved in less regular sessions. Nurses, social workers, occupational therapists and physiotherapists that have come to work with us have all attracted students from their own disciplines and are very actively involved in teaching. Much of this work involves cross pollination with other services and is very rewarding. Yet our sense of satisfaction is some-times tinged with sadness, for, whilst at grass roots level there is a real sense of pleasure derived from sharing interest and skills, there is little recognition of this at higher levels of professional organisation. Work with the elderly continues to be ranked as unskilled and undeserving of specialist status. Perhaps the next 20 years will see a change in this.

Research. New development invariably unearths new information, yet the effort of creation may not leave time or energy to collect this information. With the encouragement of the Regional Health Authority computer centre we have established a simple case register which allows us to monitor our evolution with relatively little difficulty.

In addition our awareness of the remarkable overlap in function between local authority residential homes and hospital long-stay wards became an early focus for investigation (Wilkin and Jolley, 1978). From these humble beginnings quite a large research programme has developed. This is important, not merely for the information it yields but also for its potential in gaining and sustaining interest in work within our own service and those services related to it.

Perspective

The advantages of specialised teams developing psychogeriatric services have been widely canvassed and have face validity that awaits objective evaluation. Our experience confirms that of others in finding that opportunism is a necessary additive to the recognised planning procedures and that *ad hoc* initiatives obtain remarkable improvements in the use of unpromising facilities.

Sharing experiences through the Royal College of Psychiatrists Section of Old Age Psychiatry and the British Geriatrics Society has already been used to great advantage. Yet there are clear indications from this shared experience that further developments are needed to meet logically the requirements of mentally, physically and socially impaired old people. It is doubtful if the continued division of services into geriatric, psycho-geriatric and social services should be sustained. A major realignment to create health and social services for the elderly would probably be beneficial and economically sound. Certainly there is a need to system-atise recently acquired knowledge and to encourage good practice by academic studies and training courses for nurses, social workers, physiotherapists and occupational therapists as well as doctors. In particular the naive assumption that competent professionals from such a range of disciplines will form a cohesive team without equally professional management skills should no longer be held.

References

Clarke, M., Hughes, O.H., Dodd, K.J., Palmer, R.L., Brandon, S., Holden, A.M. and Pearce, D. (1979). 'The elderly in residential care: patterns of disability'. *Health Trends*, 1, 11, 17

DHSS (1970). *Psycho-Geriatric Assessment Units.* Circular H.M. (70), 11

Hunt, A. (1978). *The Elderly at Home.* HMSO, London

Jolley, D.J. (1976a). 'Evaluation of a psychiatric service based in a district general hospital'. *International Journal of Mental Health*, 5, 3, 22

Jolley, D.J. (1976b). 'Psychiatrist into Psychogeriatrician'. *British Journal of Psychiatry.* News and Notes. November, 11

Jolley, D.J. (1977). 'Hospital in-patient provision for patients with dementia'. *British Medical Journal*, 1, 1335

Jolley, D.J. and Arie, T. (1978). 'Organisation of Psychogeriatric Services'. *British Journal of Psychiatry*, 132, 1

Jolley, D.J., Kondratowtz, T. and Brocklehurst, J.C. (1980). 'Psychogeriatric out-patient clinic'. Paper presented to Spring meeting, British Geriatrics Society, Isle of Man

Kay, D.W.K., Beamish, P. and Roth, M. (1964). 'Old Age mental disorders in Newcastle-upon-Tyne'. *British Journal of Psychiatry*, 110, 146 and 668

Kidd, C.B. (1962). 'Misplacement of the Elderly in hospital'. *British Medical Journal*, ii, 1491

Lewis, A. (1946). 'Ageing and Senility: a major problem of psychiatry'. *Journal of Mental Science*, 92, 150

McKeown, T. (1976). *The Modern Rise of Population.* Edward Arnold, London

McKeown, T., Mackintosh, J. and Lowe, C.R. (1961). 'Influence of age on the type of hospital to which patients are admitted'. *Lancet*, i, 818

MacMillan, D. (1960). 'Preventive geriatrics'. *Lancet*, ii, 1439

Pitt, B. (1974). *Psychogeriatrics.* Churchill Livingstone, Edinburgh

Post, F. (1978). 'Then and Now'. *British Journal of Psychiatry*, 133, 83

Robinson, R.A. (1962). 'The practice of a psychiatric geriatric unit'. *Gerontologia Clinica*, 1, 1

Roth, M. (1955). 'The Natural History of mental disorder in old age'. *Journal of Mental Science*, 101, 281

Sainsbury, P., Costain, W.R. and Grad, J. (1965). 'The effects of a community service on the referral and admission rates of elderly psychiatric patients', in *Psychiatric Disorders in the Aged*, W.P.A. Symposium, Manchester, Geigy

Wattis, J., Wattis, S.E. and Arie, T. (1980). 'Who are the Psychogeriatricians and what do they do?'. Paper presented to Spring meeting, British Geriatrics Society, Isle of Man

Wilkin, D. and Jolley, D.J. (1978). 'Mental and Physical impairment in the elderly in hospital and residential care'. *Nursing Times.* Occasional papers 74, 29, 117-24

Wilkin, D., Mashiah, T. and Jolley, D.J. (1978). 'Changes in behavioural character-istics of elderly populations of local authority homes and longstay hospital wards'. *British Medical Journal*, 2, 1274

11 A GERIATRIC ORTHOPAEDIC UNIT

R.E. Irvine

The orthopaedic surgeon and the physician in geriatric medicine have much to offer each other. A district where they work closely together will provide a better service, not only for the very old but for others who may need elective orthopaedic surgery.

The main opportunity for collaboration lies in the field of femoral neck fractures in elderly women, though fractures of the femoral shaft (a growing problem in the patient whose proximal femur has been strengthened by a prosthesis or an earlier fracture), other lower-limb fractures, and fractures of the pelvis and upper limbs are also of importance. In addition there is scope for collaborative assessment of patients for joint replacement.

Multiple Pathology

Multiple pathology is a cardinal feature of disease in old age. A femoral neck fracture, for example, seldom occurs in isolation. In one series 82 per cent of the patients had significant medical disability which contributed to or complicated the fracture (Thomas and Stevens, 1974). In another more than 90 per cent had problems for which the advice of the physician was of value (Campbell, 1976).

Epidemiology

Femoral neck fractures are a huge and growing problem, as people aged over 75 continue to increase in number. These fractures occur more often with advancing age and four out of five who suffer them are women. The incidence almost doubles with every five years after the age of 60 (Alffram, 1964) and in most published series 60 per cent or more of the patients are over the age of 75. Three in every hundred women over 90 fracture their femurs in one year (Gallannaugh *et al.*, 1976). There is a high mortality. Half the patients are dead in a year and a quarter become more dependent, making great demands on their families, the social services and the NHS (Thomas and Stevens, 1974).

Demand on Hospitals

The demand on hospitals can be estimated by Hospital Activity Analysis (HAA), a computerised record of the age, sex, length of stay and diagnosis of patients discharged from hospitals. In the South East Thames Region, with a population of just under 3 million, HAA showed that patients with femoral neck fractures occupied the equivalent of a 250-bed hospital throughout the year. The average length of stay for 2,619 patients was just under 5 weeks (Gallannaugh *et al.*, 1976).

HAA overestimates the numbers and underestimates the length of stay if a patient moves between hospitals in the course of one admission, as often happens with a fractured femur. In each new hospital the patient is counted again. In Newcastle-upon-Tyne transfers between hospitals were found to introduce an error of 29 per cent into HAA figures. When these were corrected by record linkage the mean length of stay for patients with femoral neck fractures was found to be 75 days, of which 48 days were spent in acute orthopaedic wards, 51 per cent of whose beds were occupied throughout the year by these patients (Evans, 1979). A similar high figure for bed occupancy by fractured femur patients was reported from Aberdeen (Smith and McLaughlin, 1974).

Hastings Figures

In Hastings 277 patients with fractured neck of femur were admitted to hospital in 1979. Women outnumbered men by six to one. The average age was 81, comparable to that of other series. Their average stay in the orthopaedic wards was 14 days compared with Newcastle's 48 and their total hospital stay averaged 38 days compared with Newcastle's 75. Moreover they occupied 30 per cent of the orthopaedic beds, not 50 per cent as recorded in other series. This lower bed occupancy by fracture patients allows the department latitude to develop a programme of joint replacement for which demand continues to grow. Joint replacement can be regarded as an important form of preventive geriatric medicine.

Principles

These results flow from principles first outlined many years ago (Devas and Irvine, 1963; Devas, 1964) and more recently developed in *Geriatric Orthopaedics* (Devas, 1977).

Age

The first principle is that no patient is too old to be denied the relief of pain and the improvement in mobility that may be expected to follow surgery. Only those who are likely to die within a day or two should be regarded as too ill for operation. There is thus no selection of patients. They come to surgery at the next routine operating session and there is an orthopaedic list every weekday. Surgery is sometimes briefly deferred for severe heart failure or unstable diabetes, but in general, delay in the hope of improving the patient's condition is self defeating. Almost all medical problems are better dealt with after operation when the patient can move without pain and nursing is easier. It is important that the anaesthetists should go along with this policy, and in Hastings they do. Nowhere, they believe, will the patient be safer than in the theatre when every breath and every heartbeat can be monitored by an expert (Haines, 1977).

Operation

The second principle is that the operation must obviate the fracture so that it can be disregarded in the subsequent programme of rehabilitation. The patient must be able to bear weight and to use the limb immediately after surgery. The McLaughlin pin and plate continues to be used for trochanteric fractures, but because of the problems of acetabular erosion cervical fractures are increasingly treated with a biarticular prosthesis, the Hastings hip, in preference to the Thompson and Austin Moore prostheses which were previously in vogue for many years (Devas and D'Arcy, 1976). Methods which do not allow immediate weight bearing or, still more, require the patient to stay in bed, are never used.

Urgency

The third principle is that there must be a sense of urgency. Speed is vital. Efforts to prevent pressure sores, for example, must begin as soon as the patient is admitted, not once the sore is threatening. Rehabilitation starts as soon as the fracture has been fixed. The longer the patient is immobile the harder it becomes for her to walk again, to dress, to cook, to resume her former pattern of life. Bedrest not only reinforces the sense of dependency, but it increases osteoporosis, predisposes to pressure sores, encourages urinary incontinence and faecal impaction and may lead to pneumonia, thromboembolism and postural hypotension.

Delay in mobilisation is not only bad for the patient, it may also mislead the relatives, who become convinced that the patient will never walk again. Her room may be given to another member of the family and her furniture is sold. Almost before she knows what has happened she has lost her place in the community and has nowhere to go. Apathy takes over and another long-stay patient has been created by mismanagement.

The Patient not the Part

The fourth principle is to treat the patient not the part. It goes without saying that the part must be managed with the utmost efficiency, but it is the patient as a whole that matters. This implies the need for a full medical, functional and social assessment: an approach familiar to anyone trained in geriatric medicine.

The Fall

It is important to learn where the patient fell. Falls in the street imply that the patient was out and about and carry a better prognosis. A fall in an old people's home carries a worse prognosis than one occurring in a private house (Devas and Irvine, 1969). The patient may find it difficult to describe how the fall occurred and the observations of a relative or neighbour may be helpful. Falls may be the presenting symptom of almost any disease in old age and are among the commonest reasons for admission to a geriatric ward. They may be classified in many ways (Overstall, 1978). One simple grouping is to divide falls into four categories (Brocklehurst *et al.*, 1978).

The most common are falls due to trips or genuine accidents with an extrinsic cause primarily, though poor eyesight may be contributory. Drop attacks form another category. These occur when the legs give way without warning and consciousness is preserved. Then there are falls due to loss of balance as may happen in ataxic conditions such as cervical myelopathy and stroke or in conditions characterised by slowness of movement like Parkinsonism. Finally there are falls associated with loss of consciousness, the epilepsies and the syncopes which have a multiplicity of causes.

Mental State

An assessment of the patient's mental state is of great value. A simple
10-point questionnaire gives a reliable and repeatable score. There are a
number of short scoring systems in use and they are probably of equal
usefulness. In Hastings we use the Mental Status Questionnaire (MSQ)
introduced from America and adapted to British use in Aberdeen (Wilson
and Brass, 1973). The mental score has proved to be an important guide
to outcome after fractured femur (Evans *et al.*, 1979). A low initial
score quite often improves after the fracture, but a persistently low
score implies dementia and a poor prognosis.

Personality

The patient's personality and emotional state are less easily quantified
than her mental score, but are also of importance. A fall with or without
a fracture is a most disturbing experience. It may destroy a person's
confidence. Some cope well and fight for their independence while
others are content to lean on anyone available.

Previous Pattern of Life

An important part of the assessment, often best gleaned from the
relatives, is a picture of the way the patient was living before the
fracture. This will give a realistic goal to aim at in the rehabilitation
programme. If it is obvious that the patient will not manage independently again, steps should be taken without delay to mobilise appropriate
support for her when she leaves hospital (Wright and Fenwick, 1978).

It is also vital to keep in touch with the relatives, to discover what
they were doing for the patient previously and what they are prepared
to offer now. The social worker is the expert in assessing how they feel
about the situation, and weighs their needs against those of the patient.

The Team

A principle very familiar to those with experience of geriatric medicine
is the need for a team. No individual can comprehend all the needs of an
elderly patient and no one is more important than the patient; neither

the surgeon, nor the physician, nor the social worker, nor the nurse, nor the remedial therapists. Each person's contribution is vital and one may have a better rapport with the patient than another, but none is self sufficient and all must work as a team. Each must respect the other's contribution and must have sufficient understanding to avoid treading on another's toes.

The team can meet in a combined ward round, or in a formal case conference or in a small ward meeting after a doctor's round. The large ward round is comprehensive and should ensure that all matters are dealt with quickly, but the number of people surrounding the patient is perhaps bewildering and the temptation for some people to have private conversations at the back of the round is hard to resist. The large case conference means a meeting away from the patient at a separate time from the ward round. The best compromise may be a ward meeting after the doctor's round, provided he is punctual and finishes his round on time, a task which some doctors find difficult.

Geriatric Orthopaedic Unit

In Hastings the accident department, the surgical admission unit and the orthopaedic wards and operating theatres are in one hospital, the Royal East Sussex, while the medical and geriatric wards are in another, St Helen's, 2½ miles away. In the early days of the NHS the geriatric wards were seen, as they often are today, as places to which other departments might offload their failures and the geriatrician was regarded as a clinical undertaker (Kemp, 1963). The arrival of a new orthopaedic surgeon in 1957 changed the situation. Mr M.B. Devas found time to visit St Helen's and met Dr L.H. Booth, physician superintendent since the days when St Helen's had been a municipal hospital under the local authority. Dr Booth and his deputy, originally the only whole-time staff, were accustomed to call in consultants from outside when they needed help and to accompany them to see the patient. So it was natural for Dr Booth, who had been left in charge of the geriatric wards when consultants appointed under the new NHS had taken over the other departments, to invite the new surgeon to see patients transferred from the orthopaedic department. Soon they began to do a regular round together and before long it was agreed that the orthopaedic surgeons should have the use of ten beds in the geriatric admitting ward, provided they visited them regularly. They were to arrange transfers to these beds without asking the physician, who nevertheless would look after the patients when they came to St Helen's. So almost by accident and quite without pain the Hastings scheme was born and continued after Dr Booth's retirement in 1958.

In 1962 a surgical ward at St Helen's hospital which had been closed for lack of staff reopened and the ten shared beds were transferred there. The geriatric department continued to provide the day-to-day care as it had always done. The ward was called the geriatric orthopaedic unit. Many years later, in 1977, the surgeons relinquished the ward to the physicians, but the geriatric orthopaedic beds remained.

Work of the Unit

The unit takes about 100 patients every year and the pattern of work has changed little. In its early days the ward was able to take about three-quarters of the women with femoral neck fractures, together with a number of people with other geriatric orthopaedic conditions. Over the past 20 years the population of the south coast of England has grown. There are now twice as many people over 75 with twice as many hip fractures as there were when the scheme started. The expertise of the surgeons has increased and more patients now go home directly from the acute orthopaedic ward. Others are discharged via a convalescent home. So now only one-third of the fracture patients, the most frail and the most ill, come to the unit, usually about a week after operation. The ward is not a convalescent unit but a place for those whose medical needs are greatest. The wealth of interesting medicine to be found in these patients is discussed elsewhere (Irvine and Strouthidis, 1977).

Discharge from the Unit

Patients stay for an average of five weeks. About 15 per cent die in the unit. The majority leave when they are fit to go home or to some form of residential care. This includes private residential and nursing homes of which there are many in Hastings and Bexhill. If any surgical problems arise requiring a second operation, the patient returns to the acute orthopaedic wards at the Royal East Sussex Hospital. Those who are not able to be discharged are transferred to the general wards of the geriatric unit after the surgical problem has been solved, their need for further treatment being determined by medical and social rather than surgical considerations. They represent about one in five of those admitted to the ward. Half of them are eventually discharged, a few more die, and the hard core of about six patients a year graduate to the long-stay wards of the geriatric unit, where half survive for over a year. In a perfect world the patient would be spared so many moves, but we have not been able to find a way to avoid them.

Nursing

The nurse allocation is the same as that for the general medical, general surgical and acute geriatric wards and normally seems adequate. The nurses qualify for the geriatric lead, an enhanced payment made to the permanent nursing staff of geriatric wards. The ward takes pupils but not student nurses. There is a part-time ward clerk.

A problem for the nurses is the high incidence of pressure sores. These almost always begin in the immediate post-operative period. The seeds are sown in the period before operation or while the patient is on the operating table. Most of the sores get better when the patient improves in mobility, but there is a need for large celled ripple beds and occasionally for a water bed. Given the money and the space a Mediscus low air loss bed would be invaluable.

Apart from equipment to deal with pressure sores the main items of furniture are those which contribute to geriatric rehabilitation. These are adjustable-height beds, preferably of the King's Fund pattern, individual wardrobe lockers so that the patient may be dressed in her own clothes, suitable chairs and a plentiful supply of walking aids. The ward also has rails in the toilets.

Shared Responsibility

A patient transferred to the geriatric orthopaedic unit comes under the day-to-day care of one of the physicians in geriatric medicine and his firm. The patient receives the same work up as is offered to other patients admitted to the department of geriatric medicine (Irvine and Strouthidis, 1977). The patient is regarded as under the joint care of the physician and the surgeon. It is a break with tradition for a patient to be under two consultants at once, but no difficulties have occurred. Each department keeps its own notes in the patient's case record. These are dictated on ward rounds and typed by the geriatric unit secretaries. The physician does a round two days before the surgeon's visit for the joint ward round. The geriatric department uses the problem-orientated system. The unit's statistics are recorded separately from both the orthopaedic and geriatric figures.

Joint Ward Rounds

The central activity of the week is the visit of the consultant orthopaedic surgeon and the joint ward round. One surgeon and one physician do the round together and the rheumatologist often attends. The senior registrars from both departments come as the round is considered an important educational experience. The pre-registration house physicians from both firms attend also. The consultants look at all the patients, irrespective of the doctors' names above the bed, and are free to make any decisions necessary. Important members of the round are the social worker, the remedial therapists and the ward sister. The round is too large for convenience, but it ensures that the whole team meet and provides the best opportunity to make certain that all the patients' problems are aired, and that nothing is overlooked which might facilitate discharge. Everyone on the round will have met the patient individually before the round and will meet her again later.

Orthopaedic Ward Visits

Apart from an emergency cross consultation the physician will not meet a patient transferred to the geriatric orthopaedic ward for a week or more after the fracture. And he will not meet her at all if she is in the two-thirds of fracture patients who do not come to the unit. This is far from ideal, but until recently seemed the best that could be achieved.

Recently, however, it has become possible for the senior registrar in geriatric medicine to do a regular ward round in the acute orthopaedic wards with the sister and orthopaedic senior house officer. This enables medical advice to be given about patients who will not be coming on to the geriatric orthopaedic unit and is felt to be an improvement. In particular there is more appropriate prescribing and better understanding when the patient is confused (Sainsbury and Benton, 1980).

Collaboration

Collaboration is the result of appropriate attitudes. Attitudes are of great importance because they determine priorities. If a surgeon and a physician wish to set up a joint scheme for a geriatric orthopaedic service, an essential prerequisite must be that they like each other and respect one another's work.

The crucial step is the decision to conduct a joint ward round. It is probably easier when only one physician and one surgeon are involved and it might be right for their colleagues to delegate this activity to them in the first instance, but the hope must be that all the staff of both departments will become involved eventually and that the juniors will take their cue from the consultants.

If the joint ward round becomes established the scheme will succeed. If it does not it will fail. A decision to hold a joint ward round is not easy to implement and it requires determination and commitment to keep it going until it becomes a habit and part of one's way of life. Established consultants have busy timetables and the longer they have been following them the more set in their ways they become. To alter an outpatient clinic or the time of a theatre list is not just a matter of a private decision. Many other people are likely to be involved and may have to be persuaded to adjust their sessions to fit the man who wants to change. In these days when every session has to be contracted for separately, few people have any spare time and the employing authority may be in difficulty if asked to fund an extra session for a joint ward round. It may well be easier for the physician to change his timetable to fit in with the surgeon, for the demands of existing clinics, operating lists and private practice are implacable. The physician must fully understand the pressures under which the surgeon organises his work and admire the skill that goes into orthopaedic surgery, while the surgeon for his part, even if he pretends that he is just a technician or 'only a humble carpenter', must become familiar with the whole-person approach of geriatric medicine (Castleden, 1977). Only a firm resolve on the part of both physician and surgeon to give the highest priority to the joint ward round will make the scheme work.

Many surgeons are not looking for genuine collaboration. They are merely hoping that someone will remove their troublesome bed blockers. No physician likes being treated like a clinical undertaker and only when he is involved early in genuine consultation will good results be achieved. This may be the reason why few schemes other than the Hastings one have been reported. Notable exceptions were those at Stoke on Trent

(Clark and Wainwright, 1966) and in South East Kent (Thomas and Stevens, 1974).

Beds

Once the decision to conduct a joint ward round has been implemented all other matters become secondary and will fall into place. This is even true of the normally thorny problem of beds. The scheme can begin by going round a number of patients wherever they happen to be. Before long it will seem tiresome to visit patients scattered through several wards, the question of grouping them together will arise, and it will seem sensible to earmark a number of beds for this purpose. These may be in the orthopaedic wards or the geriatric wards or both, as is preferred. It is more likely to be agreed that the geriatric wards shall provide beds for the scheme because the geriatric physician numbers his beds in hundreds and the orthopaedic surgeon in tens. Moreover the beds must be in a place where the geriatric firm can offer regular day-to-day care.

If the physician in geriatric medicine is able to offer the surgeon access to beds in the geriatric unit (as he will when confidence has grown up between them), he will find that he has acted to his own advantage. More patients will be discharged and fewer long-stay problems will be created.

If both departments are in a district general hospital the orthopaedic surgeon might consider the advantage of creating an acute geriatric orthopaedic ward where joint management can be offered to the patient from the beginning. This might involve regrouping the orthopaedic beds by age rather than by sex. This is not likely to be possible if the two departments are in separate hospitals.

Scale of Provision

There are no national guidelines for geriatric orthopaedics and the exact number of beds is not important. The greater the number that can be found for the scheme the greater the proportion of fractured femur patients who will be able to use them. If only the most difficult patients come to the unit, as happens in Hastings at the present time, then it will be necessary to cater for about one-third of the patients with broken hips and a provision of 0.6 beds per thousand population over 75 or 0.25 per thousand over 65 should suffice provided the length of stay in the unit is kept to five weeks. On the other hand if it was possible to plan for all the fractured femur patients, then there would be many lighter cases, the average length of stay in the unit would probably fall to about 2½ weeks and the number of beds would not have to be increased *pro rata*. The ideal would probably be a ward of 30 beds to take not only women with fractured femurs, but men also, and the range of conditions suitable for this form of management would widen.

Need for a Ward

From a clinical and nursing point of view there is nothing very special about the care of the geriatric orthopaedic patient after the first few days. The approach that is well understood in acute geriatric wards is just what is needed. These wards emphasise the need for rehabilitation concurrently with medical investigation and treatment. Special efforts are made to see the patient as a person and to understand the needs of the relatives. There is no necessity to begin with a special ward and no plans to co-operate need be put into cold storage simply because no new beds can be allocated. The success of a scheme of collaboration lies less in bricks and mortar than in the experience of working together in a joint ward round.

It is, however, a great advantage to group the patients together and if they can have a ward of their own so much the better. They must be in a hospital where there are facilities for medical investigation and for rehabilitation and where the geriatric department's junior staff can offer day-to-day care. This ought to mean a ward in the district general hospital, since an increasing number of geriatric departments have their headquarters in the DGH. What is not acceptable is to put the beds in an isolated geriatric hospital suitable only for long-stay care. To do this will ensure failure.

An important advantage of having an identified ward or block of beds for geriatric orthopaedics is that the surgeon can select the patients for transfer and send them to the unit without having to ask the physician for a bed. If these beds are considered as being separate from the acute geriatric allocation, then there is no conflict of interest when the physician is deciding on the number of admissions he can take on any day. This is an important psychological consideration when, as nearly always happens, there is great pressure for admission. In Hastings the geriatric unit takes all medical emergencies aged 76 and over and there are 1,500 to 2,000 admissions every year to a department of 260 beds.

Benefits

It is clear that the geriatric orthopaedic unit has much to offer the orthopaedic surgeon and will solve his problem of blocked beds if he is prepared to adapt his life to make it work. It is clear also that the scheme benefits the patient because it shortens his stay in hospital, though at the price of several moves during his stay. It benefits the district because it improves the efficiency of the orthopaedic service and shortens the orthopaedic waiting list without increasing beds, though not without some increase in costs. Additional prostheses, drugs and investigations, and the need for extra nurses to cope with the more intense activity of the orthopaedic wards, inevitably imply greater expenditure.

Does it also benefit the department of geriatric medicine or is it merely a device for shifting the burden from one department to another? The answer is that it is not a one-way process. The scheme benefits the department of geriatric medicine also.

In the first place the department receives a regular visit from an orthopaedic surgeon. There is thus an opportunity to discuss with an expert problems which arise every week in geriatric wards as well as in the special unit. These include patients with fractures not requiring operation, for example those of the humerus and pelvis, patients with joint problems, back pain, malignant disease and dubious radiological appearances. The combined round includes the rheumatologist, who also runs a joint scheme with the orthopaedic surgeons. With three experts available it is easier to decide the best way to help a difficult patient with his rehabilitation.

Another benefit to the department is the willing help offered when one of its patients sustains a fracture, as happens about once a month. In some hospitals deep prejudice still exists against patients from geriatric wards and it is difficult to obtain for them the investigation and treatment that would be offered without question if they came from another department. None of these difficulties arise when there is a tradition of collaboration between the two departments.

Finally and most useful of all, the scheme ensures that the physician receives his patient when something useful can be done, rather than when long-stay care is the only possibility.

Acknowledgement

It is a pleasure to acknowledge my gratitude to my colleagues Mr M.B. Devas, Mr S.C. Gallannaugh, Mr Barry Hinves, Dr Eurwen Innes, Dr T.M. Strouthidis and the late Mr Christopher Attenborough.

References

Alffram, P.A. (1964). 'An epidemiologic study of cervical and trochanteric fractures of the femur in an urban population'. Supplement to *Acta Orthopaedica Scandinavica*, 65

Brocklehurst, J.C., Exton-Smith, A.N., Lempert Barber, S.M., Hunt, L.P. and Palmer, M.K. (1978). 'Fracture of the femur in old age: a two centre study of the association of clinical factors and the cause of the fall'. *Age and Ageing*, 7, 7

Campbell, A.J. (1976). 'Femoral neck fractures in elderly women, a prospective study'. *Age and Ageing*, 5, 102

Castleden, C.M. (1977). 'Who is responsible for elderly patients in orthopaedic wards?' *Geriatrics*, 32, 65

Clark, A.N.G. and Wainwright, D. (1966). 'The management of the fractured neck of femur in the elderly female, a joint approach from orthopaedic surgery and geriatric medicine'. *Gerontologia Clinica*, 8, 321

Devas, M.B. (1964). 'Fractures in the elderly'. *Gerontologia Clinica*, 6, 347

Devas, M.B. (1977). *Geriatric Orthopaedics*. Academic Press, London

Devas, M.B. and D'Arcy, J. (1976). 'Treatment of fractures of the femoral neck by replacement with the Thompsons prosthesis'. *Journal of Bone and Joint Surgery*, 58 B, 276

Devas, M.B. and Irvine, R.E. (1963). 'The Geriatric Orthopaedic Unit'. *Journal of Bone and Joint Surgery*, 46 B, 630

Devas, M.B. and Irvine, R.E. (1969). 'The Orthopaedic Geriatric Unit'. *British Journal of Geriatric Practice*, 6, 19

Evans, J. Grimley (1979). 'Fractured femur in Newcastle upon Tyne'. *Age and Ageing*, 8, 16

Evans, J. Grimley, Prudham, D. and Wandless, I. (1979). 'A prospective study of fractured proximal femur, factors predisposing to survival'. *Age and Ageing*, 8, 246

Gallannaugh, S.C., Martin, A. and Millard, P.H. (1976). 'Regional survey of femoral neck fractures'. *British Medical Journal*, 2, 1496

Haines, A.M. (1977). 'Anaesthesia in the Elderly' in *Geriatric Orthopaedics*, M.B. Devas (ed.). Academic Press, London

Irvine, R.E. and Strouthidis, T.M. (1977). 'Medical Care' in *Geriatric Orthopaedics*, M.B. Devas (ed.). Academic Press, London

Kemp, R. (1963). 'Old age a regret'. *Lancet*, 2, 897

Overstall, P.W. (1978). 'Falls in the Elderly – Epidemiology, Aetiology and Management' in *Recent Advances in Geriatric Medicine*, B. Isaacs (ed.). Churchill Livingstone, Edinburgh

Sainsbury, R. and Benton, K.G.F. (1980). 'Medical problems in the orthopaedic wards'. *Geriatric Medicine*, 11, 64

Smith, J.A.R. and McLaughlin, J. (1974). 'A survey of fractures of the proximal femur'. *Injury*, 6, 196

Thomas, T. Glyn and Stevens, R.S. (1974). 'Social effects of fracture of the neck of the femur'. *British Medical Journal*, 3, 456

Wilson, L.A. and Brass, W. (1973). 'Brief Assessment of the mental state in domiciliary practice. The usefulness of the Mental Status Questionnaire'. *Age and Ageing*, 2, 92

Wright, W.B. and Fenwick, G.M. (1978). 'The fractured femur: why call in the geriatrician?' *Injury*, 9, 282

GERIATRIC MEDICINE AND THE COMPUTER

W.B. Wright and R.W. Canvin

In general, computers are not yet used routinely in departments of
geriatric medicine in the United Kingdom. A Medlars search produced
only one paper on the subject (Das *et al.*, 1979). Nevertheless, there are
many aspects of health care relevant to geriatricians and their departments in which the computer is emerging as a valuable tool. According
to the DHSS register of NHS computer 'hardware', there were roughly
300 computers of various capacities in the 14 regions of England in
1979.

Patient administrative systems already exist in many district hospitals,
of which the best known and most widely recognised are: Charing Cross
Hospital, London; Addenbrooke Hospital, Cambridge; the London
Hospital, Whitechapel; North Staffordshire Royal Infirmary, Stoke;
Queen Elizabeth Hospital, Birmingham; Royal Devon and Exeter
Hospital, Exeter; St Thomas's Hospital, London; and the University
College Hospital, London. There are smaller systems in a number of
other hospitals throughout the country.

Some of those major systems include the geriatric departments
where they are part of the general hospital, but in the main this is the
exception rather than the rule.

Inpatient Data Administration

A typical system, widely used in Britain and running in over 130
hospitals in Germany, is the IDA (Inpatient Data Administration) made
by International Computers Limited. This system consists of a central
computer with a number of terminals, each of which has a video display
unit and keyboard, for sending and receiving information. These terminals are placed wherever appropriate. Where necessary the visual display
can be obtained as an almost instantly produced printout.

A patient can be put on the waiting list as one of five priorities, and
each consultant can refer to a display showing his waiting list in terms
of the names, priority, sex and date entered on this list. The waiting list
can be presented as a directory of the names of patients on the list. The
computer can also show for each consultant the turnover of patients on

the waiting list, the number of additions, admissions, deletions and the average waiting time by priority. Any consultant geriatrician with central beds in a district hospital incorporating this type of computer system, will have access to this kind of printout if he wishes. This would, however, deal with only a limited number of his patients, many of whom would not be admitted to hospitals within the scheme.

The IDA system can also give an instant display of the patients by name in each ward, and show the bed state. It can show the list of patients due to be admitted to the ward and can record inter-ward transfers. The number of beds occupied and the number of available beds can also be produced immediately.

Directories of patients awaiting admission and of those recently discharged could be of considerable value to departments of geriatric medicine, where the demand for hospital services for the elderly is out-stripping the supply. These printouts could be modified to show those particularly at risk, for example. They could be used as a basis of joint discussion between community and hospital health personnel, so that these high-risk groups could have regular surveillance. The information produced on turnover and occupancy, with duration of stay per con-sultant, has limited value in practice. Most departments of geriatric medicine have a simple waiting list book or a file of cards for each patient to which they can instantly refer, and the advantages of a computerised system would not become apparent until a trained secretary had a computer terminal into which she could immediately key received information about new patients rather than entering it first on to paper files. Until the computer terminal replaces the secretary's filing cabinet, producing, as it were, a paperless office, it would be more trouble than it is worth. Nevertheless, the silicon chip is leading us into an era when the financial outlay for computer assistance will not be great and a paperless office can be considered realistically.

Outpatients

Computers have great value in the organisation of outpatient depart-ments. One such is the Nottingham system being developed by the Trent Regional Health Authority. Any geriatric service with an outpatient department in the district hospital using this system would participate. The clerk allocates an outpatient appointment using a 'clinic diary' by which the computer shows him the vacant appointments and reminds him of the booking rules. The computer will also produce an appointment letter for insertion into a window envelope, and an appointment card for follow-up appointments. If necessary, the computer can rearrange a complete clinic and print letters to advise each patient concerned. The waiting list can be printed weekly to assist in appointment selection and it can make any necessary amendments to the list which may be required by individual changes. It can print out name and address labels for each patient, thus saving a great deal of clerical work. It can produce outpatient statistics and accumulate an index of all the patients involved.

In the busy atmosphere of an outpatient department, with an almost non-stop flow of incoming telephone calls and a high amount of interrupted clerical work, the computer system is invaluable. It can reduce human error very considerably by eliminating a great deal of the repetitive and tedious elements of the work. Its ability to rearrange clinical lists according to individual changes can save a great deal of time. Where a geriatrician makes heavy use of outpatient appointments in his practice, he will reap considerable benefit from being involved in outpatient processing of this kind.

The Exeter Computer Project

The Exeter computer project is a Department of Health and Social Security funded experiment to explore further extensions of computer support to hospital and community services. It covers many aspects, some of which are already assisting the physician. At monthly intervals each specialist, including the geriatrician, receives a printout of his daily bed occupancy, admissions and discharges. He is also given the average duration of stay of his patients in comparison with the specialty as a whole. The duration of stay is displayed in figures and as a histogram which makes it possible for him to observe trends and changes in practice at a glance and to investigate these if necessary. For all specialties the admission figures, bed occupancy and duration of stay are also divided up into those aged under 65, 65 to 74 and over 74 years. This has been particularly valuable in the Exeter Health District where 20 per cent of the overall population is over 65, with resultant profound effect on the hospital and community services of almost all specialists. Using these printouts, Exeter health personnel receive regular information about the numbers of elderly patients flowing through all hospital portals. These overall histograms have been the subject of regular discussion by joint medical staff committees and the district management teams. The physicians in geriatric medicine have been appointed by their colleagues to exercise overall surveillance of the flow of elderly patients into all the major hospital departments, using these printouts, and have been given administrative assistance to do so.

The elderly population of Devon (65 and over) may increase by anything up to 50 per cent in the course of the next decade, and a number of different lines of policy are being planned to deal with this. The very fact of having information displayed for each consultant to see, which shows the number of elderly patients in his practice, is itself helpful in restricting low-priority admissions and thus preserving the overall integrity of the service.

Nursing Records

The Exeter computer project is also exploring the nursing orders system. At the Royal Devon and Exeter Hospital, in each ward where there is a computer terminal, the nursing orders have been structured so that they can be used as a working record. A series of appropriate nursing orders can be allocated for each inpatient and thus give the nurses a day-to-day display of the work required in the ward. The nurses can tell immediately how many patients require bathing, assistance with dressing, specific treatment such as wound dressing, and so on. This data base provides the potential for considerable research into planned care. The computer can elaborate a scoring system of the number of nursing procedures required in each ward and this can then be used by nursing supervisors to indicate where extra nurses are needed. It is hoped that this information will ultimately be useful in directing the flow of nurses from one part of the hospital to another, as a heavy load of nursing duties becomes apparent in an individual area. The difficulties associated with medical case notes apply also to the nursing records and there has not yet been an attempt to record information about the patient's condition from day to day on the computer.

The research potential of this development is considerable. It would be possible, for example, to work out in much clearer terms the proportion of trained and untrained nursing staff required by the different hospital wards.

This project is still at a very early stage, but there is no question about the enthusiasm of the nurses operating it. The benefits claimed include the reduction of clerical work because the computer can instantly extract diet lists, physiotherapy lists and bed states and print out as many

copies as required. Nursing officers can compare nursing orders from
ward to ward by turning to the nearest visual display terminal. It is
important to weigh these advantages against the necessity to train nurses
to enter information into the computer easily and accurately. Those
concerned feel they can overcome this difficulty. Such a system would
of course lead to a standardisation of descriptions of different nursing
duties and a more realistic appraisal of the staff required for different
types of ward. Departments of Geriatric Medicine might well benefit
from this comparative quantification of the nursing work load. New
nursing techniques and procedures can of course be made known to all
nurses simultaneously through their VDU terminal. This would probably
lead to a better and more uniform standard of practice.

Pharmacy

A highly successful aspect of the Exeter computer project has been the
delivery of information about drugs. The pharmacy department can
produce, through the computer, a virtual textbook of information on
drugs, their interactions and their side-effects, which is always up to
date and available to every practising doctor. Those doctors who do
not have immediate access to a terminal can ring up the pharmacy department, any of whose personnel can put him in touch immediately with
the latest information about drugs. This kind of information storage is
very easy for a computer. Many overseas doctors working in hospital,
and less familiar with the British Pharmacopoeia, have found this system
invaluable. It is easy to see how such a computer library can be extended
to medical and nursing procedures. The advantages of such up-to-date
information, always at hand, over the conventional handbook, which is
almost always out of date, are obvious.

Primary Care

The Exeter computer project has extended its operation to include an
urban and a rural primary care centre. These general practitioner centres
have been recording on computer all their patient notes. This is a much
more practical proposition than hospital case notes, since it involves
small entries at much less frequent intervals. These entries can be
excluded instantly from the records if they are seen to be irrelevant to
the overall care of the patient on reviewing his history. Thus only the

relevant points of history accumulate on the patient's record. General practitioners involved feel certain that they have secured better management and better patient care using the computer project. The computer keeps a record of all prescriptions that can be repeated and literally prints these out on demand by the receptionist, provided the doctor has initially authorised this. Where he has authorised the prescriptions for only a limited period, the computer automatically refuses to print repeat prescriptions. The advantage of this system to elderly people can be imagined.

Follow-up appointments are similarly dealt with by the computer. The age/sex index can produce a regular display of those elderly people who, for instance, have reached the age of 75. This makes a preventative programme and research into the value of prophylactic medication (e.g. with vitamin D in the prevention of osteomalacia) a real possibility.

It is likely that the family practitioner lists of all patients throughout the country will be filed by computer in the foreseeable future (Dendy, 1980). Using these files, lists of patients graduating to high-risk age groups could be presented on a regular basis. This would open up many possibilities of prevention which might well lead to a safer, higher quality life for the elderly in the community.

Computer-aided Diagnosis

Over 20 years ago, Ledley and Lusted (1959) considered the use of computers as an aid to medical diagnosis. Since that time some progress has been made in diagnosing specific diseases. For example, Fries (1970) in the diagnosis of arthritis, Taylor *et al.* (1972) in the diagnosis of thyroid disease, while Leaper *et al.* (1972) reported that their computer-aided diagnostic system was significantly more effective than the clinician in diagnosing abdominal pain. In geriatric medicine, the computer has been used as an index of mental status (Gedye *et al.*, 1972) and its value is being tested in the examination of cerebral blood flow (Exton-Smith, 1980). Despite these and many other individual applications, computer-aided diagnosis does not appear to have figured largely in the practice of medicine. After an extensive review of the (mainly American) literature, Fisher *et al.* (1975) concluded that it would be at least ten years before computer-assisted diagnosis has a significant impact on medicine. This was because of the technical, medical and political problems of developing and validating appropriate models and of collecting the massive amount of data required.

Planning Geriatric Services Using Computers

Deciding how to spend money on services for the elderly has always
been a difficult exercise. Like mental handicap and psychiatry, the
elderly always suffer from heavy competition from the acute services.
The government has recognised this and has attempted as far as possible
to channel money to where it is needed most. Even when money is
allocated to the elderly, there is difficulty in putting it to the best effect.
There is a clamour of competing claims for extra beds, extra hospital
and community nurses, day hospital places and community support
services. More than one budgetary purse is involved and the local expert
responsible for each form of provision is bound to feel that his service
deserves the highest priority.

To help with decision-making, various national norms have been
proposed (e.g. 10 beds per thousand aged over 65; 2 day places per
thousand aged over 65). These norms may be quite inapplicable to
individual areas or districts. They take no account of the relative
provision of existing resources. One can only make an inspired guess
at the relative effect of other provisions on the adequacy of any one
norm. Norms take no account of difference in demand. In a retirement
area there may be far more private accommodation available than elsewhere, making the norm of hospital bed provision for that area excessive.
There are many other factors peculiar to each area which make for a
different public demand for state hospital and community services,
none of which are reflected in the norm. There are no norms for new
services or innovations. Where, as is usually the case, there is rationing
of services, norms are of little help in assessing the relative effects of
equally deficient services. Where services have to be cut down, their
relation to the norm will not help to predict the effect of these
stringencies.

Increasingly, the computer is being used to try to help solve these
problems and provide a rational means of helping to plan services for
the elderly as well as other care groups. One such approach is called the
Balance of Care approach to joint planning.

Balance of Care

The term Balance of Care is really synonymous in this context with
'balance of resources'. It is concerned with planning the balance between
health service and social service resources, i.e. the balance between
hospital, residential home, day care and domiciliary care.

The Balance of Care approach to joint strategic planning is designed to help managers decide the overall allocation of key resources to the main care groups such as the elderly, the younger physically handicapped, the mentally ill and the like. It consists of two main features:

(1)   a classification that enables local professional opinion to be formulated about appropriate care for various types of patient or client in each of the care groups;

(2)   a mathematical model representing the use of different health and social resources and how they interact. The model is programmed on a computer to estimate the resource consequences of various proposed courses of action. The philosophy and mathematics of the model have been described elsewhere by Gibbs (1978).

Using the computer model, managers are able to consider one care group, say the elderly, or perhaps more usefully they can consider all the main care groups together. This enables them to examine, for example, what effect demands for extra resources for the younger physically handicapped have on the provision of resources for the elderly.

The resource consequences are measured in terms of:

1.   the amounts of each resource provided for each type of patient compared with an agreed desirable level;
2.   the number of patients of each type for whom care is to be provided;
3.   the total quantity of each resource;
4.   expenditure.

Classifying Elderly Patients

The purpose of the classification is to define each category unambiguously and in sufficient detail so that professional case workers (consultants, senior nurses, senior social workers, etc.) can propose appropriate desirable forms of care for typical patients in each category. Using data from sample surveys it must be possible to estimate the number of people in each category in the catchment population.

In Devon, the classifying characteristics of elderly patients are levels of:

physical disability
incontinence
mental state and associated behaviour disorders

social circumstances

By combining different levels of each characteristics, 32 categories of elderly patient have been defined. This classification has been developed by an advisory team of consultant geriatricians, a psychiatrist, a senior nurse and senior social services officers with responsibility for providing services for the elderly.

How Many Patients?

To find out how many patients 'in need' are in a catchment population — however those 'needs' are defined — surveys must be carried out. In the Balance of Care approach in Devon, the numbers of people in each of the defined categories currently receiving care have been estimated from surveys of people in different forms of institutional, day and domiciliary care. Surveys of the populations in the South West and elsewhere give some measure of the total number of people in each category, whether receiving care or not. One such survey was carried out by Amelia Harris (1971). Using such information, estimates have been made of the proportion of those people in each category in the population actually receiving care now. It is important to note that such surveys show considerable overlap. People in the same category receive a variety of different forms of care at present. How many will be cared for in 3 or 5 years' time? Obviously this is not known so an assumption has to be made. One such assumption is that the same proportion of the estimated population, by age and sex, will be cared for as now; this is the assumption made in Devon and whose con-sequences have been explored. Other assumptions can easily be examined by the computer; for example it may be considered that a greater proportion than now should be cared for in future to account for the present 'unmet need'.

Alternative Forms of Care

Some of the alternative forms of care will be cheaper, some more readily available than others, while some will be preferred to others; and for some there may be no expressed preferences. It is this concept of alternatives that enables the model to be used to calculate which allocation of scarce resources is 'best' within the constraints of certain well-defined rules. Constraints which are realistic in terms of local circumstances can be applied to any of the resources.

For each category of patient, a team of professional case workers proposes alternative packages of care that they consider are appropriate.

The first stage of their task is to consider the basic package, e.g. geriatric hospital or day hospital plus domiciliary services or day centre attendances plus enhanced domiciliary services, etc.

The second stage is to agree on the desirable amounts of each resource – the 'standards' of provision. An example of one set of alternatives for patients of a specified category is given in Table 12.1.

Table 12.1: Alternative forms of care considered appropriate for elderly people with moderate physical disability who are regularly incontinent at night but who have no mental or behavioural disorder: they live with others who can support them. (In this example the computer has not been allowed to place more than the existing numbers in residential or hospital care.)

Resource	Alternative forms of care and average provision per week			
	A	B	C	D
Geriatric day hospital visits	2			
Day centre visits		2		
Home nurse visits	1	1	1	1
Home help hours	15	15	19	17
Meals	0	0	0	0

The third stage is to decide whether there are any constraints to impose on each category. For example, 'the proportion of patients in category "X" to receive hospital care should be the same as at present' or 'no more than 10 per cent of patients in category "Y" should be cared for at home'.

Given a shortage of resources (the normal state of affairs), three distinct methods of rationing can be examined using the computer model:

(a)   caring for patients with acceptable levels of provision lower than the desirable standards;
(b)   applying specific limits to some of the resources;
(c)   caring for fewer patients;

or these may be combined in some way.

What is there to Prevent us Providing all the Resources Required?

Planning is dogged right at the start by such statements as 'We won't be able to afford more than ——', so a decision is made at a very early stage, without any examination of what is desirable, or any other options.

The Balance of Care approach, on the other hand, separates out the three components:

(a)   What is professionally desirable?
(b)   What is physically possible in the planning period?
(c)   What is financially possible?

The classification enables the team of advisers to specify what forms of care are professionally desirable without the constraints of what can be achieved or afforded – these constraints can all be considered at a later stage using the computer model.

Those managers responsible for planning the services are required to indicate what they think can physically be achieved in a given time span. For example if we are looking 5 years ahead, a new geriatric hospital could not be built, but perhaps 30 beds could be made available in an existing hospital with little additional capital cost. Another example is that it may be possible to increase the number of home nurses by no more than 50 per cent in that time.

An alternative approach is not to impose any physical constraints on the growth of resources, but rather to use the model to calculate what should be provided (within financial limits) and then consider whether it is feasible; and only then to impose a constraint on the appropriate resource.

Managers today are all too aware of the dangers in estimating how much revenue will be available in one year's time, let alone in 3 or 5 years hence. So the approach adopted in Devon uses the computer's ability for rapid calculations; a range of possible financial futures is examined. In this way resources, which may be indicated for expansion or contraction under different financial circumstances, are identified.

Rationing Scarce Resources

Given the above information together with information about the existing resources and their unit revenue costs, plus capital costs of additional resources, the Balance of Care model is used to calculate the consequences of the various assumptions. One such calculation obviously will not produce 'the plan' but its purpose is to generate and answer questions about the service of the 'what if . . . ?' type. In this way, new sets of assumptions are made, the consequences of which are calculated quickly using the computer model. This cyclical process is repeated until the managers are satisfied that they have explored the feasible options open to them. They are then able to produce their strategic plan, armed with the information from the results of these calculations.

One set of results of such a calculation is shown in Table 12.2 which gives the allocation of key resources to the elderly in 1977 and what they could be in 1988 under a given set of constraints and a fairly optimistic financial climate. Not surprisingly there is pressure to increase the day hospital provision, from cost considerations and a shift of policy towards community care.

Table 12.2: Example of a proposed allocation of key resources for the elderly in Devon under a given set of constraints and an optimistic financial climate

	Provision	
	1977 actual	1988 calculated
Resource	Amount	Amount
Geriatric beds acute	430	560
long stay	870	1,360
Psychiatric beds (dementia)	480	1,340
Residential home places[a]	4,950	4,950[c]
Day hospital places (geriatric & psychiatric)	220	760[b]
Day centre places	50	540[b]
Home nurse wte[d]	216	540[b]
Home help wte[d]	580	960[b]
Meals 1,000 p.a.	470	770[b]
No. of elderly people cared for	23,700	32,000

a. Includes LA, voluntary and private residential homes.
b. An overall physical constraint limited further increases in provision.
c. Constrained to be no fewer than this number as a matter of policy.
d. wte: whole time equivalent.

In this calculation, the number of residential home places was constrained to be no fewer than the existing number. However, the calculations show that they could be reduced in number. Possibly the

buildings could be used as day centres. This reduction could be achieved
by reserving them for those more seriously handicapped than at present
and providing domiciliary care for the less seriously handicapped patients.

The growth in hospital provision is perhaps surprising, but part of
the explanation lies in the projected growth of elderly people in Devon,
especially of those aged 75 and over. The projection used in this
calculation anticipated a 42 per cent increase in the 75 + age group in
Devon which accounts for much of the increased disability to be cared
for.

Subsequent calculations, following modifications to the proposed
alternative forms of care, still reflect the move from residential care to
domiciliary care, and an increase in hospital beds. This demonstrates
the general robustness of the output of the model.

One method of rationing scarce resources is to provide less than the
desirable standard of provision. Clearly it is not possible to provide part
of a hospital bed but it is possible to provide fewer than the desirable
number of meals or home nurse visits. It is up to the managers and their
advisers to decide on the standards which will be set. 'What would be
the consequences if we insisted that the quotas must all be at least 60
per cent?' would be a valid 'What if . . . ?' question to pose. The speed
with which the computer can calculate enables more options to be
examined than would otherwise be the case.

The Balance of Care approach enables the major care groups to be
considered together, so that the interactions can be readily explored.
Alternatively, a single care group such as the elderly can be examined in
considerable detail. It thereby provides a forum for the managers from
both health and social services to discuss their different viewpoints. In
this way, the Devon AHA and Social Services Department are beginning
to use the model to illustrate, for example, the resource consequences
of one authority's proposed actions, for the other. This in turn prompts
the 'What if we . . . ?' type of question that enables the managers to
explore relatively quickly the various options that might be available.

The approach is not limited to current forms of care, but it can
estimate the implications for other resources of introducing a new
resource; this has been done in examining resources for the younger
physically handicapped.

The framework of a classification linked to alternative forms of care,
forces managers and advisers (and researchers) into a more analytical
approach to planning the provision of resources. This has the advantage
of requiring that assumptions are made explicit and allows the discussions
to be more objective. Although the example given is for area planning,

the approach can be used equally well for a district or for a locality within a district, and this has been done in Devon. The speed of calculation when using the computer enables many options to be examined, which may not have been possible otherwise.

Epilogue: a Cautionary Tale

Anyone considering the use of computers in relation to geriatric department development will turn at an early stage to the concept of computer support in the analysis of routine admission data. From the very beginning of a joint psychogeriatric assessment unit in Exeter there was the opportunity of applying this support. There had been general interest for sometime in the idea of joint geriatric psychiatric reception centres for the mentally confused elderly, and some guidance had been issued by the DHSS. It was decided that a ward could be set up in a large mental hospital, which could be serviced jointly by geriatricians and psychiatrists and which would take, as far as possible, all those over the age of 65 suffering from mental disturbance of sufficient severity to demand removal from the community within a defined area.

From the outset it was felt that a great opportunity would be missed if the progress of this reception unit and its relation to the community could not be monitored in some way. The idea of a progressive computer analysis of the patients received, appealed to all those concerned and a working party was set up to define how best to use the resources. It was realised that the psychogeriatric problem was a large and growing one, and that it was specially prominent in Devon. It seemed likely that a computer supported unit could give useful information which might help other areas in the country to set up appropriate services for the mentally disturbed elderly. If the case notes for the admitted patients could be prepared in such a way as to be amenable to computer analysis, a great deal might be learned about the prognostic and management significance of certain symptoms occurring in certain types of individuals with a defined social background. The effect of early intervention and management by a jointly run unit on the geriatric and psychiatric services, and on community and local authority care, could also be measured with significant administrative benefit. It was known that only a small proportion of mentally disturbed elderly people were referred to hospital, and it would clearly be valuable to know in what circumstances such help was really necessary and what were the precipitating factors; whether, for example, the environmental factors outweighed the clinical ones. All these possible research lines could be grafted onto the ordinary function of the unit from its inception with the help of the computer.

At preliminary working party meetings the main lines of enquiry soon became clear. The prognosis and ultimate placement of elderly people admitted to this unit should be examined in relation to:

(a) What sort of people they were.
(b) What were their living conditions.
(c) What was the relative importance of mental disease, physical disease and environmental factors in precipitating referral.
(d) What was the significance of certain physical signs and symptoms in relation to prognosis.
(e) What proportion of these people were amenable to treatment.

In addition to the above, it was hoped that the value of certain non-specific therapy might be explored as time went on.

When it came to the itemisation of these ideas it became apparent that they were very complex. For example, a description of what sort of people were admitted would have to include age, sex, civil state, how long retired, present income, any change in income, usual daily activities, dietary habits, alcohol intake, drug therapy, history of previous mental and physical illness, and family history, etc.

As regards the mental and physical condition these were much more complex than the identification of the patient and his environment.

The itemisation of the required data amounted to over 50 headings, some of which included very large numbers of sub-headings, resulting in thousands of potential patient profiles. These items were pruned ruthlessly, yet it became apparent that if one was to end up with a set of case notes which described each patient in any worthwhile way, most of the 50 headings would have to remain.

As a result, it was necessary to begin the work of the unit with case notes for each patient which included over a score of pages to be filled in by the admitting medical officer. Nevertheless, there was such enthusiasm over the development of this unit, that it was decided to press on with these bulky case notes. These notes remained a source of surprise and amusement in any other departments to which patients were transferred. Nevertheless, the medical staff set to work in keeping these notes as complete as possible. Most of the items on each page had simply to be ticked off, which meant that the medical officer had hardly any writing to do, so that theoretically they might not take him any longer than writing up conventional case notes. On the other hand, to fill in these voluminous notes at the bedside was difficult; yet if they were completed away from the bedside, many items were liable to be forgotten.

As might have been expected, many items were left unmarked, especially when they were negative. This was an inevitable result of having such notes. It is difficult to imagine how, under the circumstances, this could be prevented in the ordinary routine of medical ward work. The same applied to the nursing, social work and other items. As a result many of the possible research lines originally envisaged could not be pursued.

Even so, the admissions over the first two years produced an enormous amount of data, amounting to literally piles of computer printout. In spite of having over 400 cases to examine, the numbers of individuals in each of the different categories representing source of referral, civil status, previous occupation, drug therapy, and so on, were so small that differences between groups were very often below the level of statistical significance. Worthwhile positive conclusions could not, therefore, be drawn from the great bulk of these figures. The same applied to the clinical data.

The items which involved sufficiently large groups of patients to reach significance tended to be too superficial and to establish simply what was known already – that, for example, a person living in his own home was more likely to return there than someone living in the home of a relative or friend; that people living alone were more liable to end up in a local authority home or hospital; that the diagnosis of delirium led more often to death or early recovery than the diagnosis of dementia; that greater age led to a worse prognosis, etc.

As regards the overall effect of the establishment of this unit, the destination of patients on discharge showed again what might have been expected – that there was a trend towards hostel or hospital accommodation in these patients and that half of them would not return home.

Some observations about differences in the death rate in patients with various symptoms reached significance. For example, the presence of incontinence of faeces, or severe restlessness on admission, doubled the death rate, as did a history of coma. The effect of diagnosis only reached significance when the diagnosis was made on the widest terms, though it could be seen that the expected trend of a high incidence of bronchopneumonia and urinary infection among these admissions was confirmed, and that malignancy was not an important factor among these confused patients.

After two and a half years the computer study came to an end and it was apparent that the enormous amount of work which had been put into computerised case notes had yielded small reward.

A great number of lessons were learned from this exercise. The computer analysis of diagnosis or prognosis in relation to mental disturbance or physical symptoms, as an on-going routine, is not as yet a practical possibility unless a few particular hypotheses are being tested. Each hypothesis must first be thought out in the simplest terms and one must resist the tendency to test a variety of related possibilities. It must be certain that the required data will be collected routinely and faithfully recorded for as long as necessary, and one must be careful to aim at producing information that will be of practical rather than theoretical value.

On the other hand, the flow of admissions, the source of referral and the age, sex and civil state of patients admitted can all be collected and displayed as required. Information about the patients discharged may be even more useful. In Exeter an attempt is being made to collect this information using the same structure as in the Balance of Care project. Thus as a decision is made to discharge an elderly patient from hospital, his continence, physical independence, mental state and social support are graded simply, and the supporting services that are being arranged for him are recorded. This information will be used as an on-going local check on the relevance and accuracy of the estimations made by advisers for each category of disability in the development of the Balance of Care approach to planning. However, as can well be imagined, this information could also be the basis of a high-risk register to which community physicians and nurses could refer when planning the deployment of services and personnel. The case conference system for making decisions about discharges lends itself readily to the collection of such information.

References

Das, S.K., Anderson, J. and Kataria, M.S. (1979). 'Geriatric Medicine; Model for Computer Oriented Research Analysis'. *Journal of the American Geriatric Society*, 1, 27
Dendy, P.R., SMO, DHSS (1980). Personal communication.
Exton-Smith, A.N. (1980). Personal communication
Fisher, L., Kronmal, R. and Diehr, P. (1975). 'Mathematical Aids to Medical

Decision-making', in *Operation Research in Health Care – A Critical Analysis*, Shuman, L.J., Speas, R.D. Jr. and Young, J.P. (eds.). The Johns Hopkins University Press, Baltimore

Fries, J.F. (1970). 'Experience Counting in Sequential Computer Diagnosis'. *Archives of Internal Medicine*, 126, 647

Gedye, J.L., Exton-Smith, A.N. and Wedgwood, J. (1972). 'A method of measuring mental performance in the elderly'. *Age and Ageing*, 1, 74

Gibbs, R.J. (1978). 'The use of a strategic planning model for Health and Personal Social Services'. *Journal of the Operational Research Society*, Vol. 29, 9, 875

Harris, A. (1971). *Handicapped and Impaired in Great Britain*. HMSO, London

Leaper, D.J., Horrocks, J.C., Staniland, J.R. and de Dombal, F.T. (1972). 'Computer-assisted diagnosis of Abdominal Pain Using "Estimates" provided by Clinicians'. *British Medical Journal*, 4, 350

Ledley, R.S. and Lusted, L.B. (1959). 'Use of Electronic Computers to Aid in Medical Diagnosis'. *Proceedings of the Institute of Radio Engineers*, 47, 1970-7

Taylor, T.R., Shields, S. and Black, R. (1972). 'Study of Cost-Conscious Computer Assisted Diagnosis in Thyroid Disease'. *Lancet*, 2, 79

13 ESTABLISHING NEW SERVICES: CANADA AS A CASE STUDY

D. Robertson

Canada, with territory approaching ten million square kilometres, is the second largest country in the world. Three-quarters of its 24 million people live in urban centres and the majority of the population lives in southern Canada in a strip 4,000 kilometres long and 200-300 kilometres deep. The density of population of the country as a whole is 2 per square kilometre as compared with 231 per square kilometre in Great Britain. The country is a confederation of ten provinces, each with its own provincial government, and two territories which enjoy some degree of local autonomy.

In 1967, the centenary year of Canadian confederation, over one-half of Canada's population was 25 and under. It was not until 1971 that the elderly in Canada exceeded 8 per cent of the population, thus making the country an 'old country' as defined by the World Health Organisation. Population projections indicate a growth of the proportion of citizens over 65 from 8.1 per cent in 1971 to over 12 per cent by 2001, although some provinces are close to this proportion already.

There will be a disproportionate growth in the number of very elderly, and in particular of very elderly women in Canada. Projections for the year 2031 indicate an over 300 per cent increase in the over 85s, while the general population will increase by only 66 per cent. Clearly, special health care services for the elderly are necessary to meet present needs and will be required to meet anticipated future needs.

In the previous chapters, the issues involved in establishing a geriatric service have been addressed. While the most complete network of medical services for the elderly is to be found in the United Kingdom, special health care programmes for the elderly have been developed in the last decade in Canada, the United States, Australia and New Zealand. In this chapter the special considerations involved in establishing a geriatric service in Canada will be outlined. The principles of medical care of the elderly differ little between the UK and Canada, however the practical application of these principles is greatly influenced by differences in the structure of the health care delivery system and by differences in the programmes designed to meet the needs of the elderly.

Health Care Delivery in Canada

In Canada, in the early 1980s, we cannot speak of a single health care delivery system. Under the British North America Act of 1867, responsibility for medical services, with certain minor exceptions, rests with the provinces. This contrasts with the United States of America, where Medicare and Medicaid are federally funded and administered programmes and where a national health insurance system is under consideration.

A brief account of the Canadian health care delivery system will be given in order to provide a background against which the special issues concerning the elderly may be viewed. The names by which facilities caring for the elderly are known differ between Canada, the United States and the United Kingdom and these various names for corresponding 'levels of care' are shown in Table 13.1.

Prior to the Second World War, Canadians requiring professional health care services or admission to hospitals were responsible for the cost of these services. The employed, the fit and the young could obtain insurance against part or all of the cost of hospital or outpatient services through private insurance carriers, but the unemployed, the chronically sick and the aged were uninsurable by group plans and were served either by a municipal doctor system or by the 'public' outpatient and inpatient services of larger hospitals.

A provincial hospitalisation plan was instituted in Saskatchewan in 1948, with other provinces following in the 1950s and 1960s. Saskatchewan then introduced the first provincial medical care insurance plan in 1962 and the controversy surrounding the introduction of this plan led to a partial withdrawal of medical services for 23 days – the first 'medical strike' in North America. Following federal funding initiatives, other provinces instituted medical care insurance plans in the late 1960s and early 1970s, so that by 1972 residents of all provinces of Canada were covered by provincially organised medical care insurance schemes. These programmes apply to all residents of each province with the exception of special groups such as native people and veterans of the armed services who are entitled to additional or alternate federally administered services.

Within each province one or more government agencies administer hospitalisation insurance, medical care insurance and prescription drug plans, and reimburses facilities and practitioners based upon an agreed *per diem* rate or on a schedule of fees. In some provinces a premium is paid by an individual or head of a family while in others the

Table 13.1: The Federal classification of levels of care and common names of facilities for the elderly in Canada, and their equivalent in UK and USA

Classification of Levels of Care (Canada)	Canada	UK	USA
1	Cottages, courts, etc. (often associated with nursing homes)	Sheltered Housing	Intermediate-care facilities
	Homes for the aged, lodges, personal care homes	Part III accommodation Sheltered Housing	Skilled nursing facilities, Nursing homes
2	Nursing homes, personal care homes, special care homes	Part III accommodation Long-stay wards in geriatric units	
3	Extended (continuing) care hospitals, chronic care hospitals, personal care homes, auxiliary hospital, psychogeriatric wards or hospitals	Long-stay wards in geriatric units, slow-paced rehabilitation wards in geriatric units, psychogeriatric wards in hospitals	Skilled nursing facilities, chronic hospitals
			State mental hospitals
4	Special rehabilitation wards and centres	Active rehabilitation	Rehabilitation centres of hospitals
5	Acute care hospital (for patients of all ages)	Acute medical and surgical wards of general hospitals, Assessment wards of geriatric units	Acute general hospitals

hospitalisation and medical care plans are funded through general revenues or by the proceeds of a retail sales tax. In provinces where premiums are levied, the aged and the unemployed are exempt.

Provincial hospitalisation plans cover the use of standard ward accommodation and the cost of surgical operations and prescribed drugs while in hospital. Private insurance is available to cover the cost of private rooms and special nursing. While some provinces charge the user a small *per diem* rate, it would be true to say that the entire Canadian population, regardless of age, has access to a fully insured hospital system.

Most physicians practising in Canada operate on a fee for service basis. A physician performing an inpatient or outpatient service may bill the patient or the provincial paying agency for the cost of the service based upon a schedule of fees published by the provincial medical association, or negotiated between the provincial association and the paying agency. When a patient is billed directly, the patient is reimbursed the approved cost of the service by applying to the paying agency. Some physicians and surgeons bill in excess of the rates which have been negotiated in their province, a practice known as 'extra billing'. In this circumstance the patient is responsible for the difference, and while the sums involved are usually small, extra billing is of particular concern to the poor and the elderly.

There is no Canadian equivalent of the British family practitioner's 'list'. While many patients continue to consult one physician over a period of many years, at any time a patient may consult any other primary care physician or specialist and it is not uncommon for a patient to be under the care of several physicians. In addition to a referral practice, some specialists practise primary care, some for a wide range of problems, and others for primary care problems related to their area of specialisation.

Most physicians, whether specialists or family physicians, divide their working day between their private offices and one or more hospitals. Many are members of the medical staff of one or more hospitals in their community. In cities where patients have a choice of several hospitals, often based on religious or cultural preference, the family physician will require privileges to practise in several hospitals in order to attend his patients who present 'out of hours' at the hospital emergency department and who may require admission. Although some physicians continue to see 'out of hours' patients in their offices or on house calls, the majority of primary care at night and on weekends is conducted in the hospital emergency department.

Recognition of the role of the family physician within the health care system is essential to an understanding of the special considerations in establishing a geriatric service. In addition to privileges in an acute hospital, where he may admit patients to medical, paediatric, obstetric and surgical services and perform certain surgical procedures, the family doctor will often have admitting privileges to chronic care facilities and to nursing homes.

Health Care and the Elderly Canadian

As in other Western countries, the elderly in Canada use medical and hospital services with disproportionate frequency. For example, in Saskatchewan, a western Canadian province with a population of one million persons, of whom 11 per cent are over age 65, the elderly utilise 42 per cent of hospital days, 23 per cent of all insured medical services and 30 per cent of prescription drugs.

When an older person suffers an acute uncomplicated illness, or a complex breakdown in independent living, he is usually admitted to an acute medical ward where he is cared for by a family physician and/or specialist. In teaching hospitals interns and residents will participate in his care; however in smaller hospitals and in rural areas there are no junior medical staff. When, after a period of inpatient care, he cannot easily be returned to his own home, application may be made for admission to an extended-care hospital or nursing home, and rather than returning to his own home to await placement, he will very likely remain in the acute hospital for months or years until he is transferred.

The elderly living in the community may be in their own home, living in highrise public housing, or, less commonly than in Britain, living with family members other than their spouse. Community services designed to keep the elderly in the community, such as day hospitals and social day programmes, are few. At present about 12 geriatric day hospitals are in operation in Canada, and with the exception of programmes in British Columbia, Manitoba and Saskatchewan, home care services are similarly underdeveloped. Lack of co-ordinated home care and community support services, long waiting lists for admission to extended-care facilities, and the comparative ease of entry into acute hospitals, has led to acute hospital admission as the usual response to even minor breakdowns in health or the capacity for independent living.

In the acute hospital the elderly share facilities with younger, less disabled patients. The elderly person who remains on an acute ward for a long time soon develops unnecessary functional dependency, induced, in part, by an environment which is not conducive to maintenance of self-care skills and independence. A potentially remediable breakdown thus leads to an apparent need for institutionalisation.

In contrast to the ease of entry into acute hospitals, entry into extended-care hospitals and nursing homes requires screening and may involve a wait of months or years either at home or in an acute-care bed. In most provinces the cost of care in an extended-care hospital is insured and in some this extended-care benefit also applies to nursing homes, although in some provinces the cost to the patient of nursing home care exceeds the monthly pension income by a considerable margin. No one is denied entry to a nursing home on a basis of inadequate funds as provincial social service departments will assure payments to a nursing home in case of need. However, a serious problem arises when one of an elderly couple requires admission to a nursing home and joint assets must be liquidated and used to pay the cost of care.

While there are regional differences in the rates of institutionalisation of the elderly in Canada, it is generally held that the elderly are about twice as likely to be institutionalised in Canada as in Great Britain or the United States. The actual institutionalisation rate of the elderly depends upon whether only those who are presently in long-term care facilities are counted, or whether those occupying acute care beds awaiting transfer to extended-care facilities are included. In the latter case an institutionalisation rate of around 10 per cent is present.

In some provinces special services are available to former residents of psychiatric facilities or to patients who have developed psychiatric illness in old age. Some provinces, for example Saskatchewan, have integrated former psychiatric patients who could not be returned to the community into long-term care facilities used by patients without psychiatric illness. Other provinces, for example Ontario, have separate systems of clinics, hospitals and nursing homes for the acute and long-term management of psychiatric illness in the elderly.

Special groups, such as North American native people and veterans of the armed forces, are eligible for special treatment through federally funded and organised programmes. The Department of Veterans' Affairs now maintains few acute general medical and surgical hospitals for the population which it serves, but continues to provide extended care and domiciliary care, or hostel accommodation.

Special Health Care Services for the Elderly Canadian

There are presently a dozen or so specialists in geriatric medicine practising in Canada, most of whom have obtained their training in geriatric medicine, if not their training in internal medicine, in the United Kingdom. Three or four residents are now training in geriatric medicine programmes in Canada. Within the foreseeable future an examination for a certificate in geriatric medicine will be open to fellows of the Royal College of Physicians of Canada who have trained in internal medicine and have special training or experience in geriatric medicine. It is reasonable to suppose that within the next decade or two every Canadian university will be able to attract a nucleus of three or four specialists in geriatric medicine whose function it will be to teach undergraduates and postgraduate trainees, practise in a model geriatric unit and conduct clinical research.

Having so few specialists distributed over so wide an area, and bearing in mind the interprovincial differences in the organisation of health care services, it is not surprising that widely divergent specialty services have developed. Rather than catalogue existing specialised geriatric medicine services in Canada, five different 'models' will be described briefly. These include the free-standing geriatric assessment unit in acute hospitals, the integrated geriatric hospitals with services ranging from crisis admission to terminal care, the extended-care facility incorporating domiciliary and extended care, the assessment and placement service and the geriatric services of the Department of Veterans' Affairs.

Short-term Assessment and Treatment Units

A recent development in health care delivery to the elderly in Canada has been the development of geriatric assessment units in general hospitals. At present three units are in operation and several others are planned, particularly in the province of British Columbia where it is proposed to open ten such units. Established units exist in Winnipeg, Vancouver and in Saskatoon, Saskatchewan – the latter unit will be described as an example of such centres.

Geriatric Assessment Unit. A Department of Geriatric Medicine was established in the University Hospital, Saskatoon, Saskatchewan, in July 1978, and a temporary geriatric assessment unit opened in 1979. In the summer of 1980, a unit comprising an 18-bed inpatient assessment unit and 20-place day hospital was opened in University Hospital.

The Geriatric Assessment Unit (GAU) is a short-term facility admitting elderly patients for periods of three to four weeks. The majority of patients are admitted directly from the community at the time of breakdown in health or independent living, and where possible patients are returned to the community with appropriate home care and family support. While some patients remain in the unit for rehabilitation for periods of up to six weeks, the unit does not operate extended-care beds, nor does it have any special access to extended-care facilities in the community. Admission and discharge policies have been developed to prevent an accumulation of patients waiting for transfer to extended-care beds. When patients are admitted to the unit from other hospitals or long-term care facilities, it is on the understanding that after a period of assessment and rehabilitation the patient returns to the referring unit to await extended-care placement, if necessary.

The department is a demonstration or model unit which has a major teaching role in undergraduate and postgraduate training. Patient care activity is closely monitored to determine the desirability of establishing similar units elsewhere in the province.

Integrated Geriatric Medicine Programme in a General Hospital

St Boniface General Hospital in Winnipeg, Manitoba, provides a good example of a comprehensive geriatric medicine service within a general hospital. A similar unit is planned for the Youville Hospital, Edmonton, Alberta.

The Department of Geriatric Medicine in St Boniface Hospital was established in 1974 in a newly constructed 200-bed, five-floor extension to the hospital, in which all elements of a comprehensive geriatric service were housed. The building was originally designed as a long-stay unit of five floors, each with 40 beds. With the intention of developing an integrated geriatric service, the first medical director established several sub-programmes and allocated approximately one-third of the bed complement to extended care or terminal care. Nearly one-quarter of the beds were designated rehabilitation beds and a smaller number allocated to a crisis admission programme and intermittent and holiday relief admissions. A small geriatric day hospital was opened on one of the wards by using space designed for inpatient use (Skelton, 1978).

A medical staff of full-time and part-time physicians provide a comprehensive geriatric service ranging from assessment to long-term care within the same hospital. St Boniface General Hospital serves the community of St Boniface and is one of the teaching hospitals of the University of Manitoba. While it is unusual to find extended-care beds in a university affiliated acute-care hospital, St Boniface is not unique. A geriatric unit of extended-care beds within an acute-care complex is being developed at the University of Western Ontario in London, Ontario.

In centres where geriatric units are developed in acute-care hospitals without extended-care beds, it is desirable to establish an affiliation with extended-care hospitals and nursing homes to facilitate patient movement and to provide student exposure to the older patient in settings other than the acute hospital.

Integrated Long-term Care for the Aged

The Baycrest Centre for Geriatric Care in Toronto, Ontario, comprises the Jewish Home for the Aged (376 residents), Baycrest Hospital, which is a nonsectarian chronic care and rehabilitation hospital (154 patients), and a day care service.

Baycrest Centre seeks to provide a continuum of care for the frail, sick and dependent elderly. Community outreach is achieved by affiliation with community-based services such as the Coordinated Services to the Jewish Elderly and by a day care service which accommodates up to 300 members per week. Residents of the Home for the Aged or of Baycrest Hospital who require acute care may be treated in a four-bed medical concentrated care unit in Baycrest Hospital, or if acute hospital care is required they may be transferred to Mount Sinai Hospital. Thus, by the physical proximity of levels of care 1, 2 and 3 (see Table 13.1), and by close association with an acute-care hospital, a continuum of services is provided for the elderly 'in care'.

There are a number of examples of this concept in Canada, though none is as well developed as the Baycrest Centre. In other parts of the country apartment buildings for the elderly have been built in close proximity to nursing homes (levels 1-2). While these apartment complexes are for senior citizens only, and the rents are subsidised to the point where residents pay no more than one-quarter of their income, they do not, as a rule, contain the supervisory and care components found in sheltered housing. The older person whose capacity for self maintenance in an apartment is impaired, is transferred to the nursing home, and in most centres patient movement is, regrettably, unidirectional.

Assessment and Placement Services

The need for an assessment and placement service (APS) for patients entering long-term care may not be immediately apparent to the reader familiar with a geriatric service responsible for all long-term care of the elderly within a defined geographic area. The placement function of assessment and placement services resembles that of the Bed Bureau which secures acute hospital beds for patients in larger British cities. It differs in that long-term care rather than acute-care admission is arranged.

Where assessment and placement services do not exist, entry into long-term care at levels 1 and 2 (nursing homes and homes for the aged) is a haphazard affair. Individual nursing homes or homes for the aged maintain their own waiting lists and set criteria for admission. An individual, or a family, seeking admission of a family member may encounter considerable frustration in having to approach the admissions officer of each facility, having to determine admission requirements and complete several application forms.

In the region of Hamilton-Wentworth, Ontario, which has a population of 413,000, of whom around 10 per cent are over age 65, there are 7 acute care hospitals, 393 chronic care beds, 1,106 nursing home beds in 15 different facilities, plus 150 beds for patients discharged from psychiatric hospitals. There are, in addition, 6 homes for the aged which, in addition to accommodating the ambulant elderly, have 441 bed-care places. While a similar situation obtains in many other areas, it was in Hamilton-Wentworth that the first comprehensive assessment and placement service in Canada was established.

Founded in 1971 by the local district health council, the district assessment and placement service now has a staff of one administrator, three registered nurses, and two secretaries, with medical and psychiatric consultants available when necessary. All admissions to the chronic care hospitals in the Hamilton-Wentworth region and approximately 90 per cent of admissions to private and voluntary nursing homes are processed by the APS.

Assessment is carried out by the patient's personal physician and by one other person. For applicants living in their own homes this other person may be a public health nurse; or for applicants in hospitals, a member of the ward team — a nurse, therapist or social worker may be involved. The completed assessment forms are screened by the APS staff who may request further information, make visits or refer patients for consultation with specialists in geriatric medicine or psychiatry. Approximately 2,500 people are referred annually and 1,074 were placed in 1980, of whom 750 persons were on the active caseload at any one time.

The Hamilton model differs from the other two models described in that it focuses on assessment for and placement in long-term care facilities and does not assess need for home care services. Recently established programmes in Manitoba and British Columbia incorporate assessment for and provision of a spectrum of services ranging from home support services to extended-care hospital.

In 1974 the Office of Continuing Care was established in Manitoba, with regional offices in each of the province's eight health regions. People may be referred for home care or extended care by a health professional or a member of their family. All applicants for extended care are assessed by a panel who review application forms completed by physicians, health professionals and family members to determine whether a home care service can maintain a disabled older person in the community. Where home support services are insufficient to maintain community placement, the panel determines the appropriate level of care.

A provincial long-term care programme was established in British Columbia in 1978. This is administered by the Ministry of Health and, like the Manitoba continuing care programme, incorporates long-term care and home care services. Individuals are assessed on a comprehensive assessment form by an assessor (or case manager) who may be a registered nurse, occupational therapist or medical social worker. The assessor reports to a local health unit team which decides on the extent, place and type of service. Where possible patients will be maintained in their own home with home support services ranging from homemakers and home-handyman to home nursing services. Where entry to extended-care facilities is considered desirable, the system is designed to give the client and the facility the maximum possible choice. Nursing homes no longer maintain their own waiting lists and a single waiting list is maintained by the long-term-care programme for 'opted in' facilities in that region.

The Ageing Veteran

The special provisions for eligible veterans of the armed services have been mentioned. At the end of the Second World War a chain of acute and long-term-care hospitals was in operation for the exclusive use of eligible veterans. Since the advent of provincial hospitalisation and medical care plans, the Department of Veterans' Affairs (DVA) has transferred the ownership of some of its hospitals to universities or to major hospital corporations. Some hospitals continue to be operated by the DVA, for example Deer Lodge Hospital in Winnipeg, Manitoba, which provides an excellent example of an integrated geriatric service for eligible veterans. Other hospitals, for example Sunnybrooke Hospital, Toronto, have been transferred to universities but continue to provide extended care for the veteran population.

Deer Lodge Hospital. The first integrated geriatric service incorporating assessment, rehabilitation and long-term care was established in Deer Lodge Hospital, Winnipeg. An admission assessment ward for veterans coming into long-term care was established in 1964-6, and in 1968 an integrated geriatric unit for the use of eligible veterans was established. There are presently around 240 beds, of which 20 are acute beds and 20-30 are reactivation and assessment beds.

A geriatric day hospital operates seven days a week and serves approximately 50 persons each weekday and 25 persons each weekend day. Patients using the geriatric day hospital are eligible for provincial home care services where necessary, and a liaison nurse operates within the day hospital.

In addition to its pioneering role in geriatric medicine in Canada, this hospital provides an excellent example of thoughtful renovation of an older building to accommodate the needs of older disabled residents.

Sunnybrooke Hospital. This former DVA hospital was transferred to the University of Toronto in 1966. The inpatient geriatric service, of some 400 beds, is for the exclusive use of eligible veterans. Within this bed complement, 45 beds are allocated to each of assessment, rehabilitation and psychogeriatrics. In addition to the hospital beds, a unit of 130 beds exists for individuals who require limited or no medical or nursing services, but who require accommodation in a sheltered environment.

While the inpatient service is for the exclusive use of veterans, approximately 25 per cent of the outpatient and 20 per cent of the day hospital patients are from the general population.

Community Assessment of Eligible Veterans. A system of community assessment of elderly veterans is planned, but has not yet been implemented. An assessment team consisting of a DVA counsellor, one health professional, a senior treatment medical officer and administrator or entitlement officer will assess veterans who are living in the community when requests are made for long-term care. Extensive use will be made of provincial home support systems to avoid institutionalisation where possible; however the DVA will probably continue to provide care in established levels 1-2 special care homes.

Establishing a Geriatric Service in Canada

It is clear that the British geriatric unit, responsible for a geographic catchment area and containing all assessment, rehabilitation, extended-care beds and day hospital places for the elderly in that area, has no counterpart in Canada. In establishing a geriatric service the task is to integrate special programmes or services into an established system which has excellent facilities for acute care of the young and middle aged but which has not yet made allowance for the special needs of the elderly.

Which programmes or services develop depend upon many factors including perception of need, other services which are already in operation and local demographic or geographic factors. The elderly are distributed unevenly between and within provinces and while many elderly people are urban dwellers, the proportion of older persons in rural areas and small towns is in some places in excess of 25 per cent. The low density of population and the great distances between larger urban areas will affect the way in which we develop specialised health services for the aged. The family physician, particularly in rural practice, will continue to provide the majority of ambulant care, acute hospital care and long-term care of the aged. Geriatric services, such as improved and co-ordinated home care services, community relief services and assessment and placement services, need to be developed on a province-wide basis and physicians and other health professionals will need training to assume leadership roles in implementing such services. In larger urban centres, and particularly in university teaching hospitals, departments of geriatric medicine operating short-term assessment, rehabilitation and treatment units will provide a referral service and educational resource for training physicians and other health professionals.

Home Care Services

Three of ten Canadian provinces either have, or will soon have, a co-ordinated system of home care including homemaking services, home nursing, therapy services, medical social worker, meals-on-wheels and home handyman services. In other provinces some of these services, particularly home nursing and meals-on-wheels, may be obtained directly by the patient. In one other province, Ontario, home care services are available on an 'acute' basis, which is rarely suitable for the elderly, although 'chronic' home care services have been subjected to pilot study in a number of centres and may be available on a permanent basis in the future.

Co-ordinated home care services are being developed through provincial departments of health or social services, or their equivalents, and provide access to a spectrum of subsidised services through a single contact. There are obvious client advantages in this approach compared with an unco-ordinated situation where an older person or his family must attempt to arrange services through a variety of agencies at full cost. Province-wide subsidised home care brings with it the need for assessment of need, monitoring and evaluation and accountability for expenditure.

Standards of performance need to be set, pre-employment training and staff development programmes must be established, and special consideration needs to be given to the problems of service delivery in remote rural areas where it may be difficult to attract and retain trained staff.

The physician in geriatric medicine will not be involved in the day-to-day operation of home care services but will be consulted when new programmes are developed, as some 70-80 per cent of home care clients are elderly.

Community Relief Services

Home care services are but one component of the spectrum of services required to maintain the disabled elderly at home. A range of services from social clubs to day hospitals and psychogeriatric day hospitals need to be developed in parallel with improvements in home care. Home care, no matter how intensive, cannot provide the relief from strain which supporters of dependent patients experience with day programmes and with planned intermittent relief admissions.

Approximately 12 geriatric day hospitals were operating in Canada in 1980 and without exception these are in larger cities. A few day centres or day centres for the disabled based in nursing homes or extended care hospitals are also in operation. Even where such programmes are in operation public awareness of these programmes and of their ability to maintain frail or disabled older persons in the community, is limited. Similarly, the concept of planned intermittent readmission to relieve strain of a patient's supporters is not one which has wide understanding or acceptance by the public or the health professionals. The family supporters of the physically or mentally disabled older person are likely to cope up to the point of irremediable breakdown when acute- or extended-care admission is sought.

It is unlikely that any impact will be made upon high rates of institutionalisation of the elderly without recognising and supporting those who care for the physically and mentally disabled older person at home, in short – supporting the supporter. Any community-oriented geriatric service will need to promote the development of day programmes which provide socialisation and relief as well as more therapeutically-oriented day hospitals. Intermittent respite or relief admissions to relieve strain on a patient's supporters or to permit caring relatives to take vacations, which have been instituted on a limited scale in Saskatchewan and Manitoba, are worthy of more extensive use.

Assessment and Placement Services

The role of assessment and placement services in Canada has been discussed. Where assessment and placement services are not in operation, entry into long-term care is haphazard and assessment of the need for entry into long-term care particularly at levels 1 and 2 is based on need as perceived by employees of privately operated but partially government funded nursing homes.

As with home care services, assessment and placement services are likely to be developed by provincial government or by local health boards. The specialist in geriatric medicine will not be involved in the day-to-day operation, but is available for consultation in the design and operation of the service. Assessment and placement services need to operate in parallel with geriatric units in acute hospitals where more detailed assessment can be provided in complex cases, or where rehabilitation or day hospital treatment can be offered.

A common assessment of individuals who appear to need either long-term care or home care services, such as in British Columbia's Long Term Care Programme, where a single assessment by an independent team of assessors can establish patient needs and place the patient and his family in contact with appropriate services, may be applicable to other provinces.

A New Role for the Long-term-Care Facility

As community services, home care services and sheltered housing are developed in Canada, and as assessment and placement services more thoroughly screen applicants for long-term care, it seems inevitable that the patients cared for within extended-care hospitals and nursing homes will become both older and more dependent. In provinces without separate provision for elderly persons with psychiatric illness, the nursing home and extended-care hospital will increasingly be called upon to accommodate persons with chronic brain failure (dementia). At present in the province of Saskatchewan approximately 70 per cent of

patients in extended-care hospitals exhibit chronic brain failure
(dementia) (Robertson and Rockwood, 1978). In nursing homes this
condition varies in prevalence between 30 and 50 per cent, depending
on the admission policies of the institution.

The extended-care hospital or special-care home of the future will
need to be designed, staffed and programmed to accommodate the
changing needs of its residents. As in the other areas outlined above
there is an immediate challenge for the operators of nursing homes and
boards of extended-care hospitals to meet the changing needs of their
residents and to reach out into the community with day programmes
which may maintain future residents of extended-care facilities in the
community for longer periods. It is here that the family physician with
an interest in the elderly can play a role in improving the quality of
life of his older patient.

Geriatric Assessment and Treatment Units in Acute Hospitals

While most acute hospital care of the elderly patient will continue to
occur on the general medical and surgical floors of acute hospitals, the
demonstration or model assessment and treatment unit has a useful
educational role to play within larger hospitals. In order to meet present
and future educational needs and to provide centres of exemplary
patient care, it is likely that such units will develop in most teaching
hospitals over the next decade.

Federal guidelines for geriatric units in Canadian hospitals have been
published recently by the Department of National Health and Welfare
(1979). Geriatric units of 20 beds serving an elderly population of
10,000 or a total population of 100,000, depending upon demography,
geography and the existence of other programmes within the region,
have been recommended. A handful of such units were in operation in
1980. This development seems to hold the greatest promise for improving the quality of care of older people in acute hospitals. It gives
undergraduate and postgraduate trainees the opportunity of participating
in multidisciplinary assessment and management planning for the care
of older persons who present with acute illness or whose capacity for
independent living is compromised.

Where such geriatric units are established, admission and discharge
policies should be clear and the decision on admission and discharge
must remain with the specialist in geriatric medicine or the medical
director of the unit. In short-term units, the potential for blocked beds
is very real, especially in areas where the interval between acceptance
for long-term care and entry into long-term-care facilities is a matter of

months or years. Linkage with extended-care facilities is desirable to maintain patient flow through the unit.

Education of Health Professionals

Because of the diffusion of responsibility for the community and hospital care of the elderly between family physician and specialist, the developing geriatric service should provide exemplary care of the aged and act as a teaching centre for medical students and physicians in training and for other trainee health professionals.

The specialist in geriatric medicine in Canada usually has a university appointment and works either in a university teaching hospital or in facilities affiliated with universities. With two exceptions each Canadian medical school offers some teaching in gerontology and geriatric medicine which may range from the elective programme available in some schools to the one-week mandatory clinical rotation for third-year students at the University of Saskatchewan. Residents in a two-year family medicine programme should spend some time attached to a geriatric unit, although it is still uncommon for residents training in other specialties to rotate through a geriatric medicine service.

The newly qualified physician entering practice in the 1980s will encounter many more aged and very aged patients. The responsibility for medical care of an increasingly elderly population will fall not only on the family physician and internist, but also on the psychiatrist, the ophthalmologist and the orthopaedic surgeon. In addition to ensuring that all medical undergraduates receive training in geriatric medicine it is important that the content of postgraduate training curricula in the medical and surgical subspecialties includes training in the special features of diagnosis and management of older patients. Similarly didactic and supervised clinical training of nursing, therapy and other health professional students in the health problems of the aged need to be incorporated into university and college curricula.

In Canada, the specialist in geriatric medicine, or physician with an interest in the elderly, presently has the opportunity of influencing the development of medical and social services for the elderly in his region or province. While some programmes are provincially funded and apply to an entire province, the location of day hospitals, day centres and geriatric assessment units will be influenced by local considerations, one of which is the availability of physicians willing to assume a leadership role. For the physicians wishing to establish a geriatric service the availability of beds in a particular hospital, the interest shown by the boards of trustees of an institution or the availability of funding for a programme which has been initiated by a provincial government will determine the type of service which develops.

References

Department of National Health and Welfare, Canada (1979). *Guidelines for Establishing Standards for Special Services in Hospitals. Geriatric Units in Hospitals, Geriatric Day Hospitals.* National Health and Welfare, Ottawa
Robertson, D. and Rockwood, K. (1979). 'Under-recognition and Under-reporting of Chronic Brain Failure (Dementia) in Long Term Care Facilities'. Paper presented at Canadian Association of Gerontology Meeting, Saskatoon, Saskatchewan, 17 October
Skelton, D. (1978). 'Department of Geriatric Medicine in a Canadian Teaching Hospital'. *Modern Medicine of Canada*, 33, 1783

TEACHING AND RESEARCH IN GERIATRIC
MEDICINE

J.C. Brocklehurst

Notwithstanding Oscar Wilde's epithet, 'Everyone who is incapable of
learning, has taken to teaching' and George Bernard Shaw's scornful,
'A learned man is an idler who kills time with study', the relationship
between teaching and learning remains so intimate that no practising
clinician can ever afford to cease being involved in doing either. We
should therefore consider our subject both in the context of the development of academic university departments with their conscious pursuit
of scholarship and also in relation to the practising physician in geriatric
medicine as he manages and develops his service and treats his patients.
The university academic department is the natural home of teaching
and scholarship, and the development of 15 academic departments of
geriatric medicine in Britain over a period of the same number of years
may be seen to mark the movement of the specialty from childhood
and puberty into early adult life.

Teaching and research together comprise scholarship. The word
derives from 'scholia', a body of notes in the margin of a manuscript,
which expounded or criticised the subject-matter. The notes were
subsequently added to by others who pondered on the contents of the
manuscript. Scholarship is therefore the building up of a body of
knowledge and criticism. It is intimately linked with libraries and books
and it is the existence of a separate and special body of medical
knowledge which allows a discipline to be characterised as a true
medical specialty. It may therefore be appropriate to begin by examining
that body of knowledge which justifies geriatric medicine as a true
specialty.

The Content of Geriatric Medicine

The body of knowledge on which the specialty of geriatric medicine is
based derives in part from gerontology (the study of ageing) and in part
from those aspects of medicine which are unique to old age. Gerontology
in turn divides itself into three main fields – the biological, social and
psychological. The last three decades have seen enormous advances

in knowledge in each of these.

The main theories of ageing divide into two groups – that ageing is programmed and that ageing is the result of the gradual accumulation of random errors in the replication of DNA. There is much experimental evidence in support of both of these groups of theories and the truth is likely to contain elements of both of them. There is now a considerable literature on the biology of ageing. It is essential to know something about this work to understand the place of ageing as a factor influencing the presentation of disease. For instance ageing may be an element in the breakdown in independent living. It underlies the altered presentation of illness in old age and it determines the way the ageing body deals with drugs. The decremental effect of ageing on cells and so on organs and the organism does not cause breakdown but predisposes towards it and makes the body's response to what may be fairly mild insults (infections, trauma, dehydration, etc.) quite different to the response of the body of the younger person.

Pathologies accumulate as people move through their life span and these may act as a factor contributing to breakdown and to the unusual presentation of illness. This multiple pathology may lead to the prescribing of multiple drugs, the risks of which are compounded by the pharmaco-dynamic effects of ageing.

Social gerontology provides the background to our ageing societies, it analyses the social effects of population changes and describes the evolution of social and medical care for the elderly and the important demographic facts upon which such care is based. Psychological gerontology describes the effect of ageing on the individual's consciousness and its relationship with his personality. It provides methods of assessment by which we may explain the mental functioning of our elderly patients. There is an overlap between social and psychological gerontology in considering matters such as the effects of retirement, bereavement and dying in old age; the implications of various types of care, questions of loneliness and dependency and role reversal between parent and child.

Diseases often present in different ways in the elderly compared to those who are younger. In particular there are four cardinal presenting symptoms of illness in the elderly, namely mental confusion, incontinence, postural instability and immobility. Other presenting symptoms like pain and fever are modified. There are well-known but poorly described syndromes such as 'cerebral arteriosclerosis' and many forms of chronic brain failure which yet await clear understanding – as do many causes of falls, and the true nature of terminal pneumonia. The list is almost endless. In addition the whole delivery of medical care to the elderly often requires special methods and special facilities.

From this sketchy and abbreviated description of the basis of geriatric medicine (for further details see Brocklehurst, 1978), let us examine teaching and research.

Education

Why Teach?

There are two reasons for teaching students about geriatric medicine and these apply whether we are considering medical students, nursing students or students in occupational therapy, physiotherapy, speech therapy, etc. The first reason is so that all those who practise in the broad realms of medicine, nursing and associated professions may understand the issues of health and illness as they affect old people and may therefore treat them completely. The second reason lies in the education of those who will specialise in the geriatric field.

Another reason for teaching which affects every physician in geriatric medicine is to enlighten public opinion and to contribute towards health education in the geographical area in which he practises his specialty. The geriatrician's role is greater than simply providing a one-to-one service for individual patients. He is also an initiator in the development of new services and the gatekeeper who sees that those services which are available are properly used by those who are in need. To accomplish these objectives most successfully requires a good deal of public education.

Who to Teach?

The teaching of geriatric medicine to medical students has developed over the last 15 years and is still undertaken in a very different measure in various parts of the country. In the 50 per cent or so of British medical schools where an academic university department is established, obligatory teaching is likely to comprise some 50 or 60 hours during the undergraduate curriculum and to be involved in some way with examinations. Academic staff will provide the major input but service geriatricians acting as honorary or part-time lecturers are also likely to be involved.

Postgraduate medical education should be the concern of every geriatrician both in relation to himself, his own staff of junior doctors and his colleagues in general practice and in related specialties. If all this teaching is to be undertaken then he must take the initiative in setting up courses either through postgraduate tutors or by his own personal effort. Such teaching may be in the lunchtime or evening sessions, during one or two weekend courses, or in residential or non-residential courses lasting for a week or longer.

Most geriatricians are likely to be involved with lecturing to pupil or student nurses, a task which needs to be carefully thought out and prepared. In Great Britain there are now standardised post-basic courses set out by the Joint Board of Clinical Nursing Studies. The panel for geriatrics of that Board produced two curricula intended not only to update nurses in matters concerning the elderly but also to encourage them to analyse what they do in their practice, to ask why they do various things and to consider improved ways in which nursing might be carried out. The aims — as in all teaching — are threefold, that is to provide knowledge, attitudes and skills. One of the post-basic courses is a 20-day course and the other a 6-month course. It is by means of these courses that the quality of nursing in geriatric wards is likely to be improved and it therefore falls to every geriatrician to stimulate the setting up of courses in his own area and, of course, for him to take part in the teaching.

Health visitors (see Chapter 9) also are key people in the delivery of medical care to the elderly — particularly in the ascertainment of un-reported illness. The syllabus for the one-year course in health visiting makes provision for learning about ageing and old people. Geriatricians in areas where health visitors are trained should take an initiative in seeing that they and their departments are involved in this teaching. The same considerations apply to other professionals associated with medicine — social workers, therapists, activities organisers, care attendants — even chaplains and architects should be exposed to the principles of the subject.

In relation to the wider public there are three major teaching forums concerned with ageing which are now well established throughout the country. These are pre-retirement courses, stroke clubs and relatives' conferences.

Pre-retirement courses, which were pioneered by the Pre-Retirement Association, are now run by adult education departments in most parts of the country. These usually consist of day release courses for workers (and often for their spouses), some 5 to 10 years before their retirement falls due. They alert these workers to the implications of retirement and provide them with a framework on which they may begin to prepare for their own retirement. There is almost always some medical input into these pre-retirement courses.

Stroke clubs have been pioneered by the Chest, Heart and Stroke Association and already may be numbered in their hundreds in Great Britain. They provide a continuity in the rehabilitation of stroke patients. By means of fellowship and education, they help patients to minimise their disabilities and their relatives to maximise their understanding. This is a recreational and educational process in which many geriatricians have taken initiatives.

Relatives' conferences (Hawker, 1964; Leeming and Luke, 1977) help relatives to come to terms with the fact that their mother or father needs continuing care from another person. These conferences also help relatives to cope with the guilt which is sometimes inherent in this situation and they show them ways in which they may assist in caring (for instance in helping with feeding, taking patients out for visits, providing entertainment, fund raising for amenities, befriending another patient in the ward who has no relatives).

What to Teach

The syllabus of courses will vary with those being taught but the main subjects are likely to be drawn from the following list.

Ageing. Demography and social implications; psychology; biology; pharmacology.

Medicine in Old Age. Cardinal presenting symptoms (confusion, incontinence, postural instability and immobility) and their differential diagnosis.
Special problems in relation to cardiovascular disease (e.g. heart murmurs, arrhythmias, problems of hypertension, sub-acute bacterial endocarditis and myocardial infarction).
Special problems in relation to the gastro-intestinal system (for instance hiatus hernia, silent gastric ulcers and silent peritonitis, diverticular disease, ischaemic colitis and colonic ectasias).
Special problems in relation to the musculoskeletal system (osteo-arthrosis and disc degeneration, cervical spondylosis, polymyalgia rheumatica and temporal arteritis and the myopathies of old age).
Special problems in relation to the endocrine system (the unusual presentation of hyper- and hypo- thyroidism, changes in diurnal rhythms, diabetes in old age).
Special problems in relation to the respiratory system (changes in lung function, emphysema and terminal pneumonia).
Special problems in relation to the central nervous system (e.g. stroke,

Parkinsonism, organic psychosis, vision and hearing).
Problems of anaemia, nutrition, infection, electrolyte disturbances, pressure sores, and leg ulcers in the old.

The Organisation of Medical and Social Care for Old People

This includes a consideration of: the structure of the geriatric service; the structure of the social services in relation to the elderly; the assessment of unreported illness and the management of long-term care.

Wider aspects of the care of the elderly which need consideration in educational programmes include the care of the dying and medical ethics; the problems of retirement and the place of voluntary organisations.

How to Teach

Having the three broad goals of education before us—knowledge, attitudes and skills—it is clear that a variety of methods may be useful for achieving different objectives.

Knowledge is acquired by listening to or reading about facts. Lectures and directed reading therefore provide the core of information. They must be attractive and within the capabilities of those being taught. As far as lectures are concerned, the lecturer must know exactly what he is trying to impart and for what reason, and should be prepared to use visual aids where appropriate.

Many other educational approaches are available to reinforce this basic knowledge, to build up attitudes and to allow the practice of skills. These include the seminar/workshop/colloquium. These overlap somewhat in their function and basically consist of a group who share their knowledge and who are led by a teacher who probes to discover where defects in knowledge lie and seeks to correct these.

Another group of methods includes the clinicopathological conference, sociomedical conference, case conferences, clinical presentations and autopsy reviews. All these methods are patient orientated and each of them is an admirable vehicle for group learning and the development of attitudes in relation to clinical practice. Bedside teaching, the classical form of teaching in medicine, is extremely important for the development of skills in examining old people and in considering their multiple problems. Bedside teaching is best if limited to groups of no more than six.

Participant teaching methods include undertaking a project or mini-thesis, journal clubs at which one or more people present articles from recent journals and are prepared to answer questions about them, and case presentations by students either at case conferences or at clinical sessions. The 'ageing game' recently described by Robertson and Brocklehurst (1982) provides an excellent learning medium for groups of 15 to 30 students at a time.

Research

Why Research?

An old saying might well be rephrased in relation to medical research — some are born researchers, some acquire the ability to become researchers and some have research thrust upon them. As far as specialist medicine in most parts of the Western world is concerned, those who do not fall into the first two categories almost inevitably find themselves at some stage in their career in the third. It is felt a good thing for budding specialists to undertake at least one research project. There are various reasons behind this pressure of which two are most important. The first is that it might give the young doctor an interest in research and so open to him a new dimension in his specialty. The other is that it gives him some insight into how research is carried out and will thereby make him more critical of research papers which he must necessarily interpret throughout his professional life. Some might add the third and unworthy although not entirely impractical suggestion that one or more publications stemming from research projects will enhance the job opportunities of a researcher and help him to stand out from his peers when it comes to competition for coveted appointments.

Of course the basic reasons for research are to advance the frontiers of knowledge within medical science and to contribute towards the alleviation of disease and the promotion of health. Without research, medicine would remain in the backwoods. With adequately funded and imaginatively directed research there is some hope that the great scourges of later life (particularly those arising from vascular disease and senile dementia) will eventually be overcome.

For the academic, research is an important and intrinsic part of his career. For others it may serve as an interest which they may enjoy throughout their lives and which may bring them the satisfaction attendant on becoming an expert in some field no matter how small. The 'spin off' of such expertise varies from the enjoyment of contributing to professional conferences to writing a thesis for a doctor's degree or publishing a monograph.

What to Research

The young physician in geriatric medicine, as he considers the way in which he may set his hand to research, may see the field as broadly dividing itself into four main parts – basic science, clinical observation, drug trials and the organisation of geriatric care. The field that he chooses will of course be influenced by his own attitudes and interests, by the time that he has available to devote to research and by the opportunities and facilities that present themselves to him.

It is often thought that basic science is for the universities and clinical observation for the service doctor but this is not necessarily true. One has only to think of some of the early experiments in basic gerontology that were carried out with the simplest equipment to realise that there are still plenty of opportunities for everyone in this field. Sheldon's measurement of sway among normal people of all ages using the simplest of apparatus (Sheldon, 1963) allowed him to demonstrate quite clearly and objectively the increase in sway which occurs with increasing age. However, much basic research does require complex apparatus which is more likely to be found in association with academic departments (for instance the whole body counter to demonstrate the handling of electrolytes with increasing age, and the rearing of colonies of ageing animals to allow lifetime studies of cellular and organ changes). The clinician with an aptitude for this type of research will no doubt be attracted towards academic geriatric medicine. In most hospitals, however, excellent facilities exist for collaborative research with biochemists or with clinical pharmacologists into the functional changes of ageing and the body's handling of drugs.

Research in social and psychological gerontology often requires no special apparatus and important findings can accrue to the imaginative worker who can define his problem and envisage methods that may be used to solve it. There is a long tradition of using clinical observation as a research method in clinical medicine. One has only to think of Sir James Parkinson's observations on the shaking palsy (Parkinson, 1817) and much more recently Shy and Drager's observation on autonomic disorders (Shy and Drager, 1960) to realise that research of this type is the very stuff of clinical medicine itself. In the field of old age there are still many apparently simple problems to be solved in which the answers may yet come from clinical observation, for instance the nature of drop attacks, the spectrum and classification of dementia and the effects of urinary tract infection. The young doctor drawn to clinical observation as a research method is well advised to select his problems from among

those which present to him frequently (and there will be many such),
to consider measurements which are simple and accessible, and not to
be hesitant in collaborating with others in sister disciplines.

The drug trial is now so much a part of clinical practice as hardly to
be regarded as a valid part of research at all. But the clinical trials of
newly introduced medications or indeed comparative trials of many of
those which have been in use for some time, are as essential a form of
research as any other. It is incumbent on clinicians to take part in such
trials for they are the only people with access to the subjects who make
such trials possible. Trials should not be confined to medications. There
are many methods of physical treatment, some new and some hallowed
of old, whose effectiveness have by no means been proved (for instance
the use of ultra-violet light in the healing of pressure sores and chronic
leg ulcers). There are also methods of assessment which may become
useful in clinical practice and which require initial structuring and
validation. The organisation of geriatric care has evolved from the
beginning on the basis of trial and experiment. The early pioneers like
Marjorie Warren and her contemporaries developed the pre-admission
assessment of patients at home as a way of dealing with apparently
impossible waiting lists. This has become such an institutionalised part
of geriatric practice that a reassessment of its efficiency is much needed
at this time. Progressive patient care, holiday admission and day
hospitals have become part of the framework of geriatric practice as a
result of experiment and as a reaction to circumstances and all of these
require review from time to time.

How to Research

Having decided on the broad problems which will form the basis of the
research, the first thing to do is to read as much about them as possible.
What is already known? What methods have been used and do the results
seem satisfactory? Is the previous work open to criticism? The classical
pathway of research is then to formulate the problem in terms of one
or more hypotheses. The object of the research is to prove or disprove
these hypotheses. At their most basic they may be quite simple, for
example 'postural sway increases in normal subjects with advancing age'.
Or this may be linked with further hypotheses, for example, 'the increase
in sway with advancing age is significantly related to progressive visual
impairment and this relationship is more than that which might be
expected simply on the basis of each being age-associated'.

The next stage is twofold – to begin a thorough literature search and
to produce an outline protocol of the various stages through which the

research is to move, of the methods that are to be used and of the time scale to be involved.

A method of recording and retrieving information should be developed, when reviewing the literature. This will probably be some method of summarising on a card each paper read and maintaining a file, together with cross indices by author (for setting out references) and by subject. It is often not possible to complete the literature survey before proceeding to the research itself.

Next, it is very useful to present a short paper at a departmental meeting or postgraduate meeting outlining all that has been learnt so far together with the plan for the research. Almost invariably additional ideas, which may provide significant contributions to the research project itself, will be carried from such a meeting. At this stage also (if not before) a statistician should be consulted. This is essential in any project which is to be submitted to statistical analysis and many problems will be prevented by discussion with a statistician at the earliest possible stage.

This protocol must go to the ethical committee of the hospital or district and before this it should be discussed with the heads of any laboratories or X-ray departments if such departments are to be involved in any of the data to be collected.

If financial support is going to be required for personnel, equipment, or the cost of additional tests (and most hospital laboratories and X-ray departments now rightly require payment for all additional work that is involved in research projects), then a proposal to a funding body is needed and this has very often to be prepared on their special pro forma. Regional health authorities provide financial grants for research projects and for most young geriatricians they would be the natural funding body to turn to. Other sources of finance in relation to ageing research are the Medical Research Council, Social Science Research Council and the British Foundation for Age Research. If funding is being sought for more than a year, realistic estimates for inflation should be included for subsequent years.

Having got through all these preliminaries, the stage is now set for the actual beginning of the experiments or collection of data. A decision must be taken, however, as to whether this will be a pilot study or whether the main study is to be embarked on immediately. A pilot study is often of great benefit as a practical test of the protocol. Funding bodies may well stipulate that a pilot project should be undertaken before proceeding to a main project.

The research itself will proceed according to its own methods. It should be reviewed at regular intervals, to monitor progress, particularly if a considerable body of data is being generated. This of course does not apply to double blind trials of drugs.

The third stage is that of collation of results, writing and presentation of papers. Wherever possible the data should be presented in a tabular form and many researchers like to prepare their tables first and write the paper around them. Before the final paper is produced for publication the research findings should be presented as a communication at the meeting of a learned society. Often it is worthwhile beginning with the regional group of the British Geriatrics Society and thereafter the paper might be given at the national meetings of that society or other relevant scientific societies. Delivering the paper will again allow criticisms and may indeed prevent pitfalls in the subsequent preparation of the paper for publication.

In planning your research do not neglect the possibility of its forming the basis of a thesis for a higher degree (MSc, MD or PhD). The acquisition of a doctor's degree is the mark of the 'complete physician'. If the production of a thesis is being considered then early consultation with the university concerned is necessary to make sure that the work is appropriate and if necessary to register for the degree. The style of the presentation of the thesis also varies from one university to another, and has to be taken into account.

Conclusion

All geriatricians should develop a teaching role if the service they offer is going to be the best possible. Not all will become researchers, but those who do will have acquired an extra dimension which at its lowest estimate will provide a lifetime professional interest and at its highest will add significantly to the development of their scientific discipline — medicine in old age.

References

Brocklehurst, J.C. (ed.) (1978). *Textbook of Geriatric Medicine and Gerontology*, 2nd. ed., Churchill Livingstone, Edinburgh
Hawker, M.B. (1964). 'The Relative's Conference'. *Lancet*, i, 1098
Leeming, J.T. and Luke, A. (1977). 'Multi-disciplinary meetings with relatives of elderly hospital patients in continuing-care wards'. *Age and Ageing*, 6, 1
Parkinson, J. (1817). *Essay on The Shaking Palsy*. Sherwood, Nealy and Jones, London

Robertson, D. and Brocklehurst, J.C. (1982). 'The Ageing Game, a New Teaching Method in Geriatric Medicine'. *Journal of the American Geriatric Society* (in press)

Sheldon, W. (1963). 'The Effect of Age on the Control of Sway'. *Gerontologia Clinica*, 5, 129

Shy, G.M. and Drager, G.A. (1960). 'A Neurological Syndrome associated with orthostatic hypotension'. *Archives of Neurology*, Chicago, 2, 511

CONTRIBUTORS

Mr D. Ainsworth, RMN, SRN, Community Nurse, Psychogeriatric Service, University Hospital of South Manchester

Dr J. Andrews, MD, Consultant Physician in Geriatric Medicine, West Middlesex Hospital, Isleworth, and Honorary Senior Lecturer, Charing Cross Hospital Medical School

Mrs L. Atkinson, MBOT T.Dip. Senior Lecturer, West London Institute of Higher Education (London School of Occupational Therapy)

Dr Richard Bailey, MRCP, Consultant Physician in Geriatric Medicine, Crawley District Hospital, West Sussex

Mr L. Billington, RMN, Nursing Officer, Psychogeriatric Service, University Hospital of South Manchester

Professor J.C. Brocklehurst, MD, MSc, FRCP, Professor of Geriatric Medicine, University Hospital of South Manchester

Dr R.W. Canvin, Director, Institute of Biometry and Community Medicine, University of Exeter, Devon

Dr D. Coakley, MD, MRCPI, Consultant Physician in Geriatric Medicine, St James's Hospital, and Associate Senior Lecturer in Clinical Medicine, Trinity College, Dublin

Professor M.R.P. Hall, MA, BM, FRCP (London and Edinburgh), Professor of Geriatric Medicine, University of Southampton, Southampton

Dr R.E. Irvine, MA, MD, FRCP, Consultant Physician in Geriatric Medicine, St Helen's Hospital, Hastings, Sussex

Dr David Jolley, BSc, MRCP, Consultant Psychogeriatrician, University Hospital of South Manchester

229

Dr J.T. Leeming, MD, FRCP, Consultant Physician in Geriatric Medicine, Manchester Royal Infirmary, Manchester

Professor J. Pathy, FRCP, FRCPE, Professor of Geriatric Medicine, University Hospital of Wales, Cardiff

D. Ring, RMN, SRN, Community Nurse, Psychogeriatric Service, University Hospital of South Manchester

Professor D. Robertson, FRCP(C), MRCP(UK), FACP, Head, Department of Geriatric Medicine, University Hospital, Saskatoon, Saskatchewan, Canada

G. Schroeder, Medical Social Worker, St James's Hospital, Dublin

Miss P. Smith, Social Worker, University Hospital of South Manchester

Dr J.S. Tucker, BSc, MB, ChB, MRCP, Consultant Physician in Geriatric Medicine, St Luke's Hospital, Bradford, West Yorkshire

Professor Eluned Woodford-Williams, CBE, MD(London), FRCP, MRCPsych, Formerly Director of the National Health Service, Health Advisory Service (England and Wales), Lately Visiting Professor Department of Geriatric Medicine, University Hospital of South Manchester

Dr W.B. Wright, MB, FRCP, Consultant Physician, Queens Hospital Geriatric Unit, Cirencester, Gloucestershire

GLOSSARY OF TERMS RELATING TO THE UK NATIONAL HEALTH SERVICE

Area Health Authorities: The Regional Health Authorities (see below) are divided into a number of Area Health Authorities (AHA). Each AHA in turn has a number of District Management Teams to supervise basic health services at a local level. There are 90 Area Health Authorities in England.

Community Health Councils: These are bodies whose broad task is to represent the views of the 'consumer' to the health authorities. Half the members are nominated by the Local Authorities, one-third by voluntary organisations and the rest by the Regional Health Authorities.

Community Physician: Community physicians are specialists in that branch of medicine which deals with populations or groups rather than with individual patients. They are experts in health care planning and administration and social and preventive medicine.

Department of Health and Social Security (DHSS): This department is responsible for the administration of the Health Service at a national level. It is also responsible for Social Security and Personal Social Services. The Secretary of State for Social Services is the head of the department and he is responsible to Parliament.

District Nurse: These are nurses who carry out general care in the home. In order to meet the special needs of certain groups of patients there has been a tendency towards specialisation in recent years. For instance, nurses may specialise in aspects such as renal dialysis, or stoma care, or rehabilitation.

Family Doctor/General Practitioner Services: In Britain, medical care is administered in the community by family doctors and in hospitals by consultants. When the family doctor has a problem needing hospital care or investigation he refers the patient to a hospital consultant. Family doctors work mainly on a geographical catchment area basis and together with the health visitor and district nurse they form the primary health care team. It is estimated that the family doctor is the first point of contact for about 90 per cent of people seeking treatment for ill-health in Britain.

Health Visitor: The health visitor is a nurse with a post-registration qualification, the health visitor's certificate. She is not engaged in practical nursing procedures but provides a health advisory service to families and individuals of all age groups. Some health visitors have developed a specialist interest and expertise in dealing with the problems of the elderly.

Local Authorities: These metropolitan and nonmetropolitan county authorities are responsible at a local level in Britain for the organisation of personal social services such as child care, domiciliary services, residential services for the elderly and care of the handicapped. Joint Consultative Committees have been created to ensure co-operation between the Local Authorities and Area Health Authorities in the planning and implementation of matters relating to health.

Nursing Officers: Individual hospital wards are under the control of ward sisters (female) or charge nurses (male). A nursing officer has a more senior position and he/she will usually be in charge of several wards.

Primary Health Care Team: This team consists basically of the family doctor, the district nurse, the health visitor, the domiciliary midwife and, in some instances, the social worker. It is becoming increasingly more common for the members of the team to work from the same premises, usually a health centre.

Regional Health Authorities (RHA): The DHSS delegates responsibility to the Regional Health Authorities (RHA). England is divided into 14 regions and each RHA has responsibility for the services in its own region and the planning and management of capital works and expenditure.

Seebohm Report (1968): This was the report of the Committee on Local Authority and Allied Personal Social Services (chaired by Frederick Seebohm) which recommended that all personal social services should be unified, including those administered by health authorities, in a new single department under the control of directors of social services.

INDEX